OUTDOOR MEDICAL EMERGENCY HANDBOOK

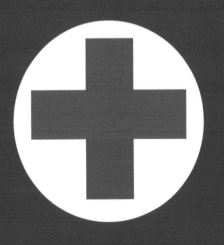

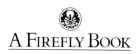

A FIREFLY BOOK

Published by Firefly Books Ltd. 2010

First printing

Publisher Cataloging-in-Publication Data (U.S.)
Briggs, Spike.
    Outdoor medical emergency handbook : first aid for travelers, backpackers, adventurers / Dr. Spike Briggs and Dr. Campbell Mackenzie.
[240] p. : col. ill. ;   cm.
Includes index.
Summary: A medical reference for traveling in potentially risky environments; includes information on all aspects of health, how to prepare for a journey, emergency response, and rescue procedures.
ISBN-13: 978-1-55407-601-7
ISBN-10: 1-55407-601-3
1. Outdoor medical emergencies.   2. Outdoor recreation--Safety measures. I. Mackenzie, Campbell. II. Title.
616.0252 dc22   RC88.9.O95B75 2010

A CIP record for this book is available from Library and Archives Canada

Published in the United States by:
Firefly Books (U.S.) Inc.
P.O. Box 1338, Ellicott Station
Buffalo, New York 14205

Published in Canada by:
Firefly Books Ltd.
66 Leek Crescent
Richmond Hill, Ontario L4B 1H1

Conceived, edited and designed
in the United Kingdom by:
Marshall Editions
The Old Brewery
6 Blundell Street
London N7 9BH
www.marshalleditions.com

Art Director Ivo Marloh
Consultant medical editor Dr. Chris Johnson
Managing editor Paul Docherty
Project editor Amy Head
Illustrators Peter Bull, Mark Franklin
Indexer Sue Butterworth
Production Nikki Ingram

Originated in Hong Kong by Modern Age
Printed and bound in China by Toppan Leefung Printers Limited

To our fellow travelers M & E
And young adventurers EFF & HFLA

OUTDOOR MEDICAL EMERGENCY HANDBOOK

First aid for travelers backpackers adventurers

DR. SPIKE BRIGGS AND DR. CAMPBELL MACKENZIE

FIREFLY BOOKS

CONTENTS

Preparation

Emergencies: How to Save and Preserve Life

Environmental Risks

Accidents and Trauma

CONTENTS Continued

Medical Disorders and Treatments

Emergency Medical Procedures

Appendices

INTRODUCTION

It is a paradox of our increasingly sedentary society that wilderness travel and adventure is rising inexorably in popularity. This is an overwhelmingly positive development. The more people who see the wonders of our world, the greater influence they may bring to bear on how we all live our lives, and perhaps our environment will be the better for it.

Such activity, however, is not without risk. As such travel becomes more accessible, more vulnerable explorers—less fit, younger and older—will venture beyond the ready reach of appropriate hospital care.

The *Outdoor Medical Emergency Handbook* provides a *vade-mecum*, literally a "take with you" ready reference book that will answer the burning question when faced with a sick or traumatized companion: "What do I do?" For the expedition medic of some experience, it will act as an *aide-memoire* for recalling medical knowledge, while reassuring and confirming that the correct action is being taken.

The handbook is suitable for all types of expeditions, from unsupported Trans Arctic marathons to family adventures. It covers ailments that may affect team members of all ages, from the very young to those older travelers who still have a thirst for adventure despite some medical "baggage."

The phrase "common things happen most commonly" applies equally to injuries and illnesses, both on land and at sea. Therefore, this handbook concentrates on the sort of simple, minor problems you are most likely to encounter and supplies the basic information on what to do, with simple, easy-to-follow illustrations on how to do it. It also gives guidance on assessing more severe illnesses and injuries, including when the casualty can be managed on location and when they should be evacuated.

Importantly, the handbook also reinforces the message that "prevention is better than cure"; anticipation of medical emergencies will avert trouble later. There is a specific section on assessing and controlling risk. Parts of this book, particularly the section on preparation and planning, contain essential information that should be read and absorbed before departure.

The team will have faith in the capabilities of the expedition leader and the medic. They will expect that the medic can get them out of immediate trouble and safeguard them for as long as it takes to either recover or reach professional help, should it be necessary. However, confidence does not always reflect competence. Therefore, it is essential that the expedition leader and the medic both obtain suitable medical training and experience.

Remember that seeking medical advice is one of the most important actions to take when faced with a difficult medical problem. A healthy team is a happy team, and above all, the ultimate goal of the expedition medic is to save and preserve lives.

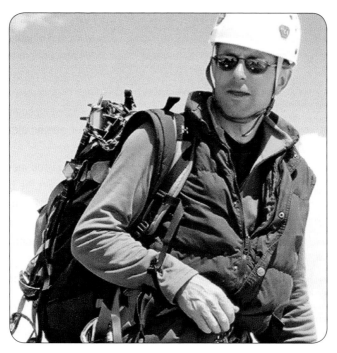

Dr. Spike Briggs

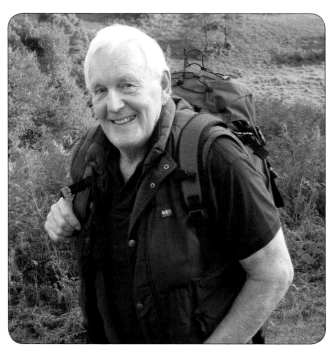

Dr. Campbell Mackenzie

HOW TO USE THIS BOOK

This book is divided into six chapters and within those into individual entries. Before you depart, read the Preparation chapter, where you will learn how to equip the expedition and prepare the medics and team members. In the wilderness, the chapter you choose will depend on the circumstances. The Emergencies, Accidents and Trauma as well as Medical Disorders and Treatments chapters will refer you to the final chapter, Emergency Procedures, for step-by-step instructions on making vital assessments, performing minor wound repair, stabilizing injuries and carrying out emergency procedures. The Environmental Risks chapter includes information specific to various settings, as well as advice on wilderness survival.

The Emergencies, Accidents and Disorders chapters all use a similar format. Within the appropriate entry, consult the flow chart for a condensed summary of evaluation and treatment. The remainder of the entry will expand on this outline, further explaining symptoms and signs, giving hints on prevention and describing the features of specific injuries and treatments.

Red boxes emphasize emergency actions

Red arrows indicate severe risks and emergency responses

Follow cross-references to further detail or to systematic instructions

Emergency procedures are explained using step-by-step illustrations

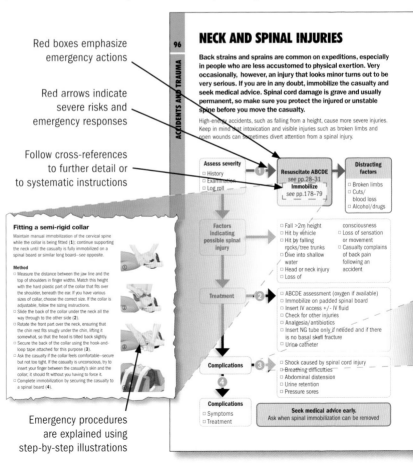

ACRONYMS AND SYMBOLS USED IN THIS BOOK

ABC	Airway, Breathing, Circulation	see p.28
ABCDE	Approach, Assess, Airway; Breathing; Circulation; Disability; Environment	see p.30
AED	Automated External Defibrillator	see p.175
AVPU	Alert; Vocal stimuli provoke response; Painful stimuli provoke response; Unresponsive	see p.182
BLS	Basic Life Support	see p.28
bpm	beats per minute	
EPIRB	Emergency Position-Indicating Radio Beacon	
GCS	Glasgow Coma Score	see p.182
IM (injections)	Intramuscular	
IV (fluids)	Intravenous	
NG (tube)	Nasogastric	
NSAIDs	Nonsteroidal Anti-inflammatory Drugs	
PLB	Personal Locator Beacon	
<	Less than	
>	Greater than	

1 History and examination

Parts of the spine

- ABCDE assessment (see pp.28-31) takes priority over everything else.
- Anyone with a head injury may well have a spinal injury as well.
- A proper examination for possible neck and spinal injuries will require a log roll (see p.177), which requires four people to turn the casualty and one to examine the back.

Cervical vertebrae (cervical spine)

Thoracic vertebrae

Lumbar vertebrae

Sacrum

Coccyx

97

NECK AND SPINAL INJURIES

Anatomical illustrations provide a guide to major parts of the body, to help you when reporting to remote medical support

Important points in the history

- How did the accident happen?
- Where is the pain?
- Are there any symptoms of nerve damage? – Numbness
  - Pins and needles
  - Loss of movement
- Any previous history of back pain or injuries?

Important points in the examination

Look Obvious injuries to head, neck, spine; swelling, bruising
Feel Tenderness, steps in spine, can the casualty feel touch and pain?
Move Can casualty move body and limbs? If neck injured, do not move it
Document Tone, power, sensation for all limbs and the main body

Quick-reference lists explain what you need to find out from the casualty and what to look for during an examination

2 Treatment

A casualty with a suspected spinal injury must be evacuated as soon as possible.
Immobilization (see pp.178-79) The whole body must be immobilized as effectively as possible using a semi-rigid collar and a padded board.
IV access and fluid Casualty may have low blood pressure and need IV fluid.
Nasogastric (NG) tube, urinary catheter (see pp.200-201) An immobilized casualty may be kept hydrated by an NG tube and will need a urinary catheter.
Analgesia, antibiotics Pain relief to settle the casualty; antibiotics for an open wound.

3 Complications

- Spinal cord damage can cause blood vessels to relax, leading to low blood pressure and shock. Seek medical advice for guidance on fluid replacement.
- Breathing difficulties may result from spinal cord injuries located high in the chest or in the neck. This is an ominous problem. Administer oxygen if available and follow ABC assessment if the casualty stops breathing (see p.28).
- The stomach may stop working, and the casualty may vomit. Insert an NG tube and aspirate the contents to reduce the risk.

4 Minor back injuries

Symptoms A minor back injury will cause localized pain that is worse on straining or coughing. Pain may extend down the leg (sciatica) and posture may be abnormal.
Treatments Administer pain relief to allow mobilization and prevent stiffness. If the casualty has sciatica, advise rest. Care should be taken with the posture during vigorous activities such as chopping wood and carrying loads.

A numbering system helps you quickly locate more detail on such subjects as complications, specific injuries or disorders and signs of severe conditions

PLANNING WILDERNESS TRAVEL

Expedition planning requires careful attention to detail and takes time, knowledge and experience. If you are deficient in any of these areas, ask for help and guidance from someone who has the necessary expertise. Planning medical resources and telemedical support is a specialized part of this process and is essential, because when you are confronted with a medical emergency, planning is over, and action must begin.

There are a number of main elements, considered below, that affect the medical planning for any expedition, whether it is a short trip in the Australian outback, a trek across the Kalahari Desert, or an exploratory expedition to polar regions.

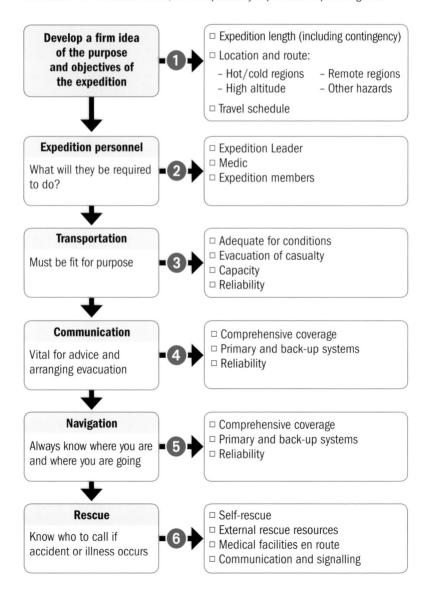

Develop a firm idea of the purpose and objectives of the expedition

1
- ☐ Expedition length (including contingency)
- ☐ Location and route:
  - – Hot/cold regions   – Remote regions
  - – High altitude   – Other hazards
- ☐ Travel schedule

Expedition personnel

What will they be required to do?

2
- ☐ Expedition Leader
- ☐ Medic
- ☐ Expedition members

Transportation

Must be fit for purpose

3
- ☐ Adequate for conditions
- ☐ Evacuation of casualty
- ☐ Capacity
- ☐ Reliability

Communication

Vital for advice and arranging evacuation

4
- ☐ Comprehensive coverage
- ☐ Primary and back-up systems
- ☐ Reliability

Navigation

Always know where you are and where you are going

5
- ☐ Comprehensive coverage
- ☐ Primary and back-up systems
- ☐ Reliability

Rescue

Know who to call if accident or illness occurs

6
- ☐ Self-rescue
- ☐ External rescue resources
- ☐ Medical facilities en route
- ☐ Communication and signalling

1 Expedition purpose and objectives

Longer expeditions to remote and harsh environments call for increased expertise within the team and additional support planning. The more remote the area to be visited, the greater the complexity of medical conditions that may require treatment. Therefore, for these expeditions, team members should be fitter, with fewer pre-existing medical conditions. Build in contingencies for unforeseen events that may significantly prolong the expedition.

Expeditions to extreme environments, whether hot, cold, high altitude or particularly remote, raise the possibility of specific medical problems that must be considered during the planning process.

Travel to high altitude and to hot and cold climates requires acclimatization. The rate of acclimatization varies between individuals, and there should be flexibility within the travel schedule to allow all team members to acclimatize fully before proceeding.

2 Expedition personnel

Routes that are particularly rigorous or remote, long distances and extreme climates require fit team members and comprehensive medical training for the medic. It is advisable, if numbers allow, to appoint two or more medics, one of whom may be the expedition leader. This provides a fall-back if one of the medics leaves the expedition or requires treatment.

All members of an expedition must be clear that the medical care they receive during the expedition is unlikely to match that of a sophisticated hospital. Certain medical conditions may endanger the whole expedition if they are not declared beforehand and proper planning undertaken.

3 Transportation

Expedition transportation may take a multitude of forms, such as trekking on foot (perhaps pulling a sled), riding horseback with pack animals or traveling in a four-wheel drive vehicle. Whatever form is used, it must be fit for the conditions. Many expeditions have turned into survival epics due to inadequate transport.

Consider, from the medical point of view, how a sick or injured team member may be transported for evacuation if they become immobile. Also, the type of transport affects the amount of medical kit that can practically be carried.

4 Communication

There has been a revolution in communication during the past thirty years. Even in the most remote parts of the globe, having a satellite telephone means that comprehensive medical advice is just a phone call away. Some forms of satellite communication also allow transmission of emails and digital pictures. Cell phones are useful, but coverage is not complete. Vehicle-mounted high frequency radios are also widely used and provide a good alternative, although satellite technology is gradually overtaking this form of communication.

There are two issues that must be considered during the planning phase, irrespective of what methods you choose. Firstly, two separate and independent forms of communication should be taken on the expedition. If carrying capacity allows, taking a high frequency radio and a satellite telephone is sensible. Two separate satellite phones will both be useless if the satellite network goes down.

Secondly, all of these mediums require a power supply: the power outlet from a vehicle engine (perhaps requiring an inverter to convert 12v DC to 110/240v AC), a solar panel (photovoltaic cells) or a large-capacity rechargeable battery with enough energy to recharge a phone several times (ideal for expeditions on foot).

For information on EPIRBs and PLBs, see p.210–11.

⑤ Navigation

It is critical to know where you are and where you are going at all times. In the event of accident or illness requiring evacuation, the rescue services will require longitude and latitude of your position, and if you are able to relay this information, it will speed up the rescue process.

The development of the Global Positioning System (GPS) in the past 25 years has significantly aided navigation, but GPS should be seen as an adjunct rather than a sole navigation system. GPS systems require power and clear sight of at least three satellites in order to function. Carry at least two GPS systems, detailed topographic maps and at least two magnetic compasses (in case one is lost).

⑥ Rescue

Even the best-prepared expeditions occasionally have to call on external rescue resources. Keep in mind that rescue operations are inherently dangerous and Search and Rescue (SAR) services should not be used unless necessary.

All available SAR services and means of contact should be identified prior to departure, together with the location of the nearest appropriate hospital care and sources of medical resupply.

Given recent advances in communications, should an accident or illness occur, the need for medical evacuation by SAR resources can be discussed with medical advisors who are familiar with these situations. Sources of advice should be identified and contacted prior to departure, so they are aware of the expedition. They may even be able to offer advice about medical planning.

Tasks before departure

Team selection

The physical and mental fitness of team members should be proportional to the arduousness and remoteness of the expedition. As part of the preparation for larger expeditions, bringing together people who are not personally known to the organizer, prospective team members may be asked to complete a medical questionnaire (see pp.214–15 for an example).

In general, any condition that may deteriorate in the wilderness to the point that it may endanger life if the casualty does not receive immediate hospital care may preclude travel to remote areas. Examples of such conditions include heart disease, diabetes, organ transplant, severe asthma and epilepsy. A review by a doctor familiar with expedition medicine may be required.

Selection of the medic

Who makes the best medic? Ideally, the person should be well motivated, and it helps if he or she has some form of medical, dental, veterinarian or paramedical background. Preferably, two medics should be appointed, in case one is injured and requires treatment. There are many training courses in wilderness medicine (*see* pp.233), and good training for the medics is essential, particularly for trips to the remote wilderness. The medics should have responsibility for reviewing the medical histories of team members and compiling the medical kit.

Immunization

All immunizations must be up to date, particularly yellow fever, for which a valid immunization certificate is required by certain countries in South America and Africa. *See* p.222 for a guide to immunization requirements.

Medical kit

The selection and quantities of drugs for the kit depends on the location, route and duration of the expedition, together with the potential requirements of the team members, depending on their medical histories (*see* pp.20–21 on the structure of a medical kit, and pp.223–25 for suggested kit contents).

Team members who take specific medicines, either occasionally or regularly, should take enough with them to adequately cover the proposed duration of the expedition, plus a contingency. It is common sense to pack the contingency supply separately to ensure the whole supply does not get lost or ruined.

Medical support

Lines of communication and sources of medical support should be in place prior to departure. In addition to government authorities, there are companies that specialize in offering telemedical support to expeditions both on land and at sea and have the technology to receive voice calls, digital images, video and email. It is helpful to discuss the nature of the expedition and the background of the team members with your medical support team, so they are fully briefed about any potential problems.

Insurance

Insurance must cover not only medical treatment but also the possible cost of rescue and repatriation, which may be considerable. Team members need their own individual insurance, and it is wise for the expedition medic to have professional indemnity insurance. However, the medic may not be covered to administer treatment in certain countries without specific insurance or to treat the citizens of certain countries wherever the expedition may be taking place.

Insurance companies may ask for the medical details of all team members, but bear in mind that disclosure to a third party requires the individual's consent.

Resupply of medical supplies

Restocking of medical supplies may be problematic, especially if the local language is not English. However, most drugs are available in most places, albeit in different packaging and using different trade names. The generic names should remain consistent around the world. You may arrange to ship resupply items from home, but this will require clear documentation and customs clearance.

EMERGENCY PROCEDURES

The maxim "prevention is better than cure" applies absolutely to the planning of expeditions to remote areas. An informed assessment of risk allows effective management of emergencies. Be proactive—anticipate adversity and plan for it.

It is said that no plan survives first contact with the enemy, and it is true that the original plan may quickly become inadequate. It is vital to prepare "in depth"—for every plan A, have a plan B. Rigid planning is best replaced by a simple, flexible format that addresses the most common medical emergencies (*see* opposite).

Managing medical emergencies is a continual learning process, and practice simulations, particularly for expeditions to remote areas, will keep the skills fresh. Every new team member should be briefed on basic emergency medical procedures.

The aim of managing medical emergencies

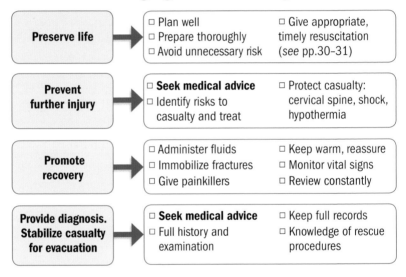

Preserve life	□ Plan well □ Prepare thoroughly □ Avoid unnecessary risk	□ Give appropriate, timely resuscitation (*see* pp.30–31)
Prevent further injury	□ **Seek medical advice** □ Identify risks to casualty and treat	□ Protect casualty: cervical spine, shock, hypothermia
Promote recovery	□ Administer fluids □ Immobilize fractures □ Give painkillers	□ Keep warm, reassure □ Monitor vital signs □ Review constantly
Provide diagnosis. Stabilize casualty for evacuation	□ **Seek medical advice** □ Full history and examination	□ Keep full records □ Knowledge of rescue procedures

Team Roles

Team Leader	Overall management and planning. In an emergency, try to avoid getting directly involved, but remain briefed on progress. Plan ahead for possible evacuation.
Medic	Assess, treat, stabilize and safely retrieve the casualty. Avoid becoming injured. Liaise and brief the team leader. Seek medical advice early.
Communication	One team member should be responsible for communication planning prior to departure and operation in the event of an emergency.
Navigation	At all times, a team member should be responsible for knowing where all members of the team are and where they are going. Transmit this information to SAR authorities.

General procedure for managing medical emergencies

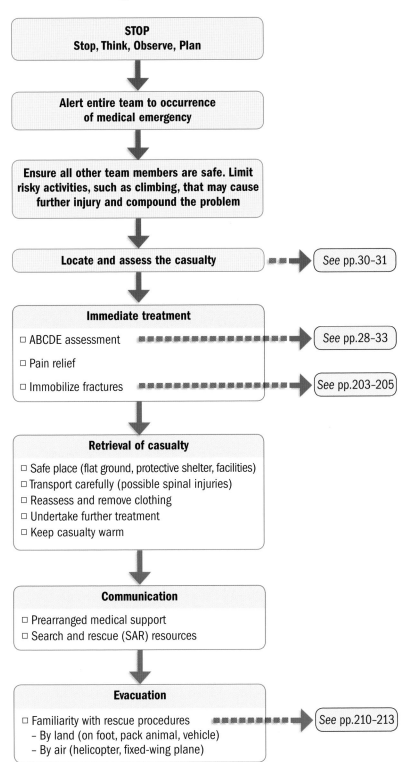

STOP
Stop, Think, Observe, Plan

Alert entire team to occurrence of medical emergency

Ensure all other team members are safe. Limit risky activities, such as climbing, that may cause further injury and compound the problem

Locate and assess the casualty → *See pp.30–31*

Immediate treatment
□ ABCDE assessment → *See pp.28–33*
□ Pain relief
□ Immobilize fractures → *See pp.203–205*

Retrieval of casualty
□ Safe place (flat ground, protective shelter, facilities)
□ Transport carefully (possible spinal injuries)
□ Reassess and remove clothing
□ Undertake further treatment
□ Keep casualty warm

Communication
□ Prearranged medical support
□ Search and rescue (SAR) resources

Evacuation
□ Familiarity with rescue procedures → *See pp.210–213*
  – By land (on foot, pack animal, vehicle)
  – By air (helicopter, fixed-wing plane)

EXPEDITIONS WITH CHILDREN

Sharing the wonders of the world with children is one of the joys of parenthood. However, this privilege comes with the responsibility of taking care of children in new environments with unfamiliar risks. This is especially the case when the child is too young to "consent" knowingly to the expedition.

The risks of physical and psychological harm can never be completely eliminated, but they can be controlled. This process involves becoming aware of the particular susceptibilities of children. It is wise to take a first-aid book specific to children and arrange medical support from advisors who are experienced in treating children.

Keeping children going

Children require proportionally more food, drink and rest at frequent, regular intervals. A tired, thirsty and hungry child will not walk far. If you modify expedition goals to take into account the child's physical and mental capabilities, this will result in a more successful and harmonious team. Boredom (in the camp, in a vehicle or on a boat) is another enemy of tranquillity and can be forestalled by thinking ahead. Carry compact games and books and provide opportunities for play and personal exploration.

A simple balance of inputs and outputs will achieve equanimity:

Inputs	Outputs
☐ Hydration (balanced solution)	☐ Opportunity for play, games, reading to relieve boredom and frustration
☐ Nutrition (tasty carbohydrates)	☐ Listen to and consider complaints
☐ Frequent opportunity for rest	☐ Frequent toileting (carry toilet tissue)
☐ Warmth in cold climates	☐ Children lose body heat faster
☐ Coolness in hot climates	☐ Children lose body fluids faster
☐ Dryness in wet climates	☐ Diarrhea and vomiting has a greater debilitating effect
☐ Reassurance and explanation of surrounding environment	

Particular risks with children

Hypothermia/heat illnesses The larger surface-to-volume ratio of children, together with less efficient thermoregulation, increases the risk of hypothermia in cold climates and heat illnesses in hot climates. Body warmth may be lost very quickly.

Communication Young children may not communicate discomfort, injury, cold, heat, thirst or hunger with the same vigor or clarity as an adult. The responsible adult must be aware of this limitation and be ready to interpret sulkiness, quietness, withdrawal and tears accordingly.

Transport Children may occasionally be carried in backpacks, on sleds or on skidoos at speed. Being inactive, they generate less body heat and may rapidly become hypothermic. Lower limbs are particularly at risk in a backpack due to constriction around the upper thigh, increasing the risk of cold injury.

Risk of injury Several aspects of a child's body make it more susceptible to injury. Small stature, flexible bones and a shorter rib cage all predispose them to increased severity of injury. Be aware of this if a child falls or is hit by a vehicle or similar. Call for medical advice immediately.

Immunizations All children should be up to date with the usual recommended childhood vaccinations. Further recommended vaccinations are listed on p.222. If you are traveling with very young children, seek specialist advice.

Infections The young immune system is less well developed, so children are more prone to infections of the throat, chest, urinary tract and skin. Young children explore at ground level with their hands and mouth, increasing the risk of infection further.

Drug and fluid dosages Doses for children are determined by weight. Medicines designed for children usually have a dosage guide on the packet. Be careful to follow the guide accurately, and do not be tempted to give more for added benefit. Do not guess or estimate dosages of other drugs. Always seek medical advice first.

Insect bites Prevention is mandatory, particularly in malarial regions. It can be tricky to persuade young children to cover up, apply repellent and sleep under undisturbed nets. Bites will feel itchy, and continual scratching may cause secondary infection. Antihistamines and hydrocortisone cream may help, but seek medical advice if itching is severe. Ticks and lice are additional risks.

Hygiene Camp showers or baths help to cool and clean hot bodies and may reduce the chance of infection.

Clothing

The standard advice for adults also applies to children, except that children are more vulnerable. Advances in clothing for children now mean that Gortex™–lined boots and shells are easily available. A triple-layer system as used in adults may also be used in children. Add an extra insulting layer in cold climates, if the child is inactive. Pay special attention to the extremities. Mitts rather than gloves keep small hands warmer. Take extras because children lose gloves regularly. "Ragg" (loop stitch) socks are available for small children and reduce the chance of blisters. Goggles and face masks may also be required.

Visibility is another factor that influences expedition clothing for children. In exposed situations, children may wander off inadvertently and get themselves into trouble. The following could be considered:

- Bright clothing with reflective patches
- Headlamps, so you can see the child in the dark and they themselves can see
- Bright life vests for inshore and marine waters, even for competent swimmers
- Whistles—teach them to blow three blasts if they are in trouble or lost.

Medical kit for children

If children under the age of twelve will be taking part in an expedition, there are additional items that should be included in the medical kit.

- Acetaminophen syrup
- Ibuprofen syrup
- Antihistamine syrup (chlorpheniramine)
- Anti-motion sickness medicines (scopolamine, meclozine)
- Antibiotic syrup (amoxicillin)
- Albuterol inhalers for wheeze
- Hydrocortisone cream

- Children's adhesive bandages
- Adhesive wound closure strips
- Skin glue
- Cold skin spray (ethyl chloride) for numbing prior to injections etc.
- Antiseptic skin spray ("dry iodine")
- Second skin spray (this may sting)
- Calamine lotion/cream

ORGANIZING THE MEDICAL KIT

The design and arrangement of a medical kit for wilderness travel is influenced by many factors, including the opinion of the medic undertaking the task. No two medics will arrive at the same solutions, but the common goal of health and safety can be achieved with markedly different kits.

There are many points to be considered in determining both the contents of the kit and the framework for organization, and these are listed below. A general inventory of suggested contents for three kit applications (base camp, field excursions and personal use) is included on pages 223–225. Additional items recommended for specific environments are included on page 85.

The medic must be involved in putting the medical kit together, so they know the contents of the kit and know how to use them. There is no point in taking a piece of equipment such as a chest drain if no one knows how to use it.

Design factors

Expertise of the medic Greater medical expertise on the expedition may justify a more sophisticated kit.

Destination Certain environments, such as malarial areas, high altitude regions, marine settings and areas of climatic extremes, entail special provision.

Remoteness/isolation A greater degree of self-sufficiency will be required in treating medical emergencies in remote areas.

Remote medical help A support team may guide the team medic in treating more complicated conditions, necessitating a more comprehensive medical kit.

Activity Specific activities such as diving, caving and ski mountaineering engender specific health risks that should be covered by the medical kit.

Size of team Generally, a bigger team requires a larger, more comprehensive kit. However, a doubling of numbers does not call for doubling the size of the medical kit. If the expedition team also includes local porters, camp staff, guides, translators etc., keep in mind that they may require treatment.

Length of trip Longer trips may require greater quantities of commonly used drugs, such as painkillers and antibiotics, but there may be an opportunity for resupply.

Previous health problems Team members may come with considerable "medical baggage" but will hopefully bring a good stock of their own medications. It is sensible to include extra doses in the kit in case there are complications.

Previous experience The experience of the team medic and of other medics that have been to the region in the past is valuable in selecting specific items for the kit.

Endemic disease Many regions that attract expeditions have endemic diseases. Think of prevention first, but treatment must be within the capability of the kit.

Transport capacity This may limit the size of the medical kit, so logistics must be taken into account. On the other hand, if a large kit is compulsory, for instance if you need oxygen for high altitude expeditions, this may dictate the kind of transport.

Economics Every expedition has a budget; larger, more sophisticated kits cost more.

Expiry date Medicines and sterile equipment have a limited shelf-life. It is wise to ensure every item has a long shelf life prior to departure—some items are manufactured with longer shelf lives than others.

Selecting medicines and equipment

Familiarity It is wise to use medicines with which the medic is familiar, unless certain conditions require specific treatments.

Infrequent side effects Using medicines with infrequent side effects will help you to avoid complicating an already difficult situation.

Controlled drugs Morphine and other similar opiates are very useful as analgesics and are often included in expedition kits. It is wise to take relevant documentation when traveling to different countries and to seek specific advice about policy in the country concerned. Keep a record of all controlled drug usage.

Multiple uses It is economic to include drugs that may be used to treat a variety of conditions (e.g. codeine—pain, diarrhea) and equipment that can be used in a number of ways (e.g. urinary catheter—chest drain, giving rectal fluids).

Storage and stability Many drugs need to be stored under specific conditions of temperature, humidity and light, losing potency if the limits are infringed (insulin becomes inactive if frozen; suppositories tend to dissolve in hot conditions, becoming a challenge to use). It is sensible to avoid medicines with strict storage criteria.

Resupply Common drugs are easier to source locally than more sophisticated drugs, which may need to be shipped from the home country (an expensive and complicated process).

Team member medicines It is sensible to continue the normal medications for team members rather than experiment with any new treatment ideas.

Arrangement of the medical kit

A medical kit may well contain several hundred items, and finding the right drug or piece of equipment shouldn't be like the proverbial needle and haystack. Organizing the kit into sections is the key.

Waterproof, airtight containers that are robust, light and compact are ideal. Lists of contents, including item expiry dates, should be enclosed in each case. It is useful to put each section in a transparent plastic pouch for fast identification.

First aid/sickness	Emergency/allergies	Painkillers
□ Cold, flu, sickness medications	□ Epinephrine	□ For mild, moderate and severe pain
□ Adhesive bandages	□ Steroids	□ Tablets, suppositories
□ Simple painkillers	□ Antihistamines	□ Injectable painkillers
□ Sunscreen	□ Sedatives	□ Local anesthetics
	□ Burn treatments	

Ear, nose, mouth, eyes	Trauma	Infections
□ Eye drops for pain	□ Splints	□ Antibiotics: 3 types, to avoid allergies; oral and injectable forms
□ Irrigation for eyes	□ Casting kits	
□ Eye bath and shades	□ Strapping	
□ Antibiotic eye/ear drops	□ Dressings	□ Antibacterial skin preps
□ Dental kit	□ Bandages	□ Antifungal preps

Skin repair	Gut	Store bag
□ Suturing kit	□ Laxatives	□ IV fluid
□ Skin stapler	□ Antidiarrheal	□ Oxygen cylinders
□ Antiseptic fluid	□ Anti-indigestion	□ Defibrillator
□ Adhesive skin tape	□ Antispasmodics	□ Reserve drugs supply
□ Skin glue	□ Rehydration salts	

ASSESSING RISK

Increased risk may lead to an increased number of injuries, which are always unwelcome but particularly so on expeditions. Injury transforms a team member from asset into liability, requiring transportation and medical care. Using control measures to avoid hazards and minimize risk increases the likelihood of expedition success and, most importantly, keeps everyone healthy and happy.

Risk assessment involves looking at all aspects of the expedition with a critical eye and identifying the hazards that may result in injury or illness if things go wrong. Once the high-risk tasks or activities are identified, control measures can be used to reduce the risk of injury.

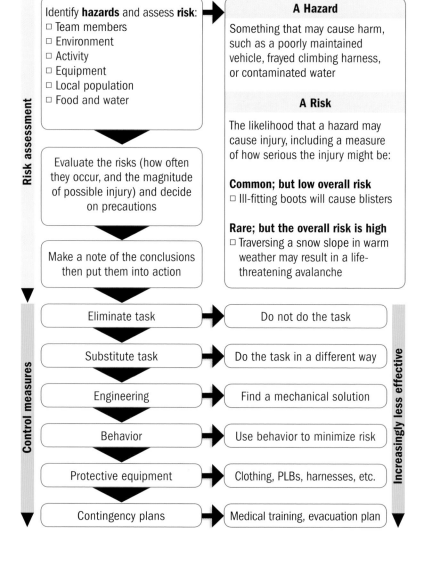

Risk assessment

Identify **hazards** and assess **risk**:
- ☐ Team members
- ☐ Environment
- ☐ Activity
- ☐ Equipment
- ☐ Local population
- ☐ Food and water

Evaluate the risks (how often they occur, and the magnitude of possible injury) and decide on precautions

Make a note of the conclusions then put them into action

A Hazard

Something that may cause harm, such as a poorly maintained vehicle, frayed climbing harness, or contaminated water

A Risk

The likelihood that a hazard may cause injury, including a measure of how serious the injury might be:

Common; but low overall risk
- ☐ Ill-fitting boots will cause blisters

Rare; but the overall risk is high
- ☐ Traversing a snow slope in warm weather may result in a life-threatening avalanche

Control measures

Eliminate task	→	Do not do the task
Substitute task	→	Do the task in a different way
Engineering	→	Find a mechanical solution
Behavior	→	Use behavior to minimize risk
Protective equipment	→	Clothing, PLBs, harnesses, etc.
Contingency plans	→	Medical training, evacuation plan

Increasingly less effective

Predicting the risk of accidents

It may be possible by knowing and recognizing the hazards present to calculate an "accurate" evaluation of risk, but risk is not black and white; it does not give a definite answer as to whether or not an accident will occur.

Hazards do not exist in isolation. The more hazards present at any one time, the greater the risk of accident. If all conditions line up and converge at one point in time, an accident will happen. This is the "Swiss cheese" model of accident causation or, to put it more formally, the "cumulative act effect." As an example, if team members are tired, don't know where they are or where they are going, the weather is worsening and it's getting dark, the risk of accident is increasing. The situation must be recognized and control measures instigated. In this instance, the STOP strategy should be employed: Stop, Think, Observe and Plan.

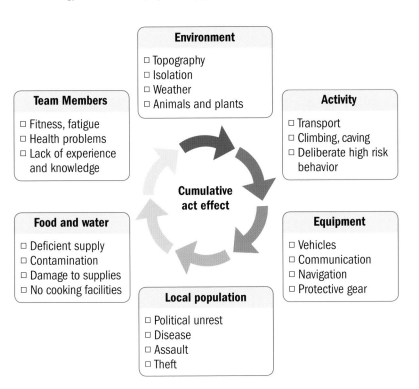

Environment
- Topography
- Isolation
- Weather
- Animals and plants

Team Members
- Fitness, fatigue
- Health problems
- Lack of experience and knowledge

Activity
- Transport
- Climbing, caving
- Deliberate high risk behavior

Cumulative act effect

Food and water
- Deficient supply
- Contamination
- Damage to supplies
- No cooking facilities

Equipment
- Vehicles
- Communication
- Navigation
- Protective gear

Local population
- Political unrest
- Disease
- Assault
- Theft

Golden rules of accident prevention

- Build a culture of safety and establish reasonable, sensible control measures within the expedition team.
- Always operate within your limits, particularly when responsible for others.
- Know how to use and regularly maintain your personal equipment.
- Consume adequate food and fluids.
- Get some sleep whenever you can.
- Avoid alcohol and drugs in the wilderness.
- Obtain knowledge and experience of where you are going.
- Maintain a good level of fitness.
- Communicate effectively and regularly.

TAKING A HISTORY FROM A CASUALTY

The first step in finding out what is wrong with an injured or sick casualty is to understand what has happened, both the immediate events and those further back in the past. This is no easy task, even in a fully equipped hospital, so is particularly difficult in the wilderness.

It is vital to remember that resuscitation and treatment of life-threatening injuries or illnesses takes precedence over a detailed history. However, a history of sorts is still absolutely necessary in emergency circumstances. The way to go about this is detailed in Assessment of a Sick or Injured Casualty (*see pp.30–33*).

It is useful to have a structure for taking a history, both for medics and nonmedics; this will minimize the chances of essential information being missed. It also helps when transmitting medical information to medical advisors, by ensuring it is logical and comprehensive. Avoid medical jargon, which may be misleading if not used correctly. It is usually impossible to get the whole history in one go; it may come together over a few hours or even days, with information from various sources, not only the casualty.

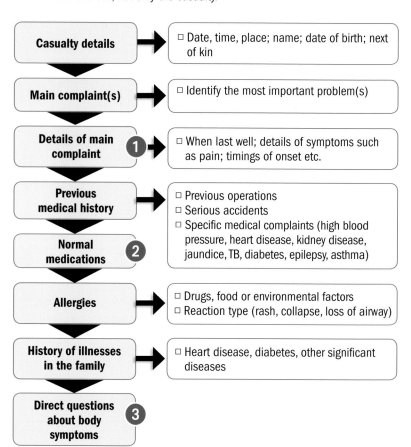

| Casualty details | → | □ Date, time, place; name; date of birth; next of kin |

| Main complaint(s) | → | □ Identify the most important problem(s) |

| Details of main complaint ❶ | → | □ When last well; details of symptoms such as pain; timings of onset etc. |

| Previous medical history | → | □ Previous operations
□ Serious accidents
□ Specific medical complaints (high blood pressure, heart disease, kidney disease, jaundice, TB, diabetes, epilepsy, asthma) |
| Normal medications ❷ | | |

| Allergies | → | □ Drugs, food or environmental factors
□ Reaction type (rash, collapse, loss of airway) |

| History of illnesses in the family | → | □ Heart disease, diabetes, other significant diseases |

| Direct questions about body symptoms ❸ | | |

① Details of main complaint

Complaint
What happened?
What is wrong now?
When did you have it last?
Do you know what it is?

When were you last well?
Have you had this before?
How long did it last?
What treatment worked last time?

Pain
Where is the pain worst?
Do you feel it anywhere else?
Is a sharp, dull, or constant?

How severe is the pain (out of 10)?
What makes it worse?
What makes it better?

② Normal medications

- Specifically ask about heart medications, inhalers, epileptic and diabetic medications, antimalarials and oral contraceptives.
- Get details of immunizations, prophylactic medications and past foreign travel.
- Also, ask about alternative medicines, homeopathic remedies, recreational drugs, alcohol and smoking.

③ Direct questions about body symptoms

ASK ABOUT:

Heart and circulation
Chest pain
Palpitations
Shortness of breath
Swelling of the ankles
Pain in the legs when walking

Lungs
Shortness of breath
Pain related to breathing
Cough
Wheeze
Sputum—amount and color

Mouth, throat and intestines
Nausea and vomiting
Indigestion, reflux
Abdominal pain
Distension
Last bowel movement—consistency
Nature of stool—color, blood
Appetite, weight loss

Kidneys, bladder and genitals
Pain on passing urine
Passing large urine volumes frequently
Color of urine
Loin pain
Discharge from genitals
Date of last menstrual period
Any miscarriages

Nervous system
Headache/stiff neck
Pain on looking at light
Visual acuity
Hearing
Seizures and fainting
Weakness or numbness in limbs

Musculoskeletal system/skin
Pain or stiffness on moving limbs
Muscle pains or swelling
Joint pain or swelling
Stability while walking
Skin diseases/problems
Allergic reactions affecting skin

EXAMINING A CASUALTY

Examinations may be particularly difficult in bad weather and poor light conditions, particularly when an injured casualty is wearing bad weather gear. It is worthwhile to plan how you would transfer an injured, immobile casualty before you have to do it.

Examination is a sensitive activity but is absolutely essential if the casualty is seriously injured or sick. The examination can be confined to the leg, if that is the only injured part, but should be comprehensive, covering the whole body (including the back) if the casualty has fallen from a height and is unconscious. It may be necessary to expose part or all of the body, depending on the extent of injury. This may be inconvenient and difficult to achieve with a sick or injured casualty and it may also be detrimental, because the casualty could become very cold while uncovered. Minimizing and making best use of exposure time is imperative. The basis for examination is **look, feel, listen, move** and compare left with right.

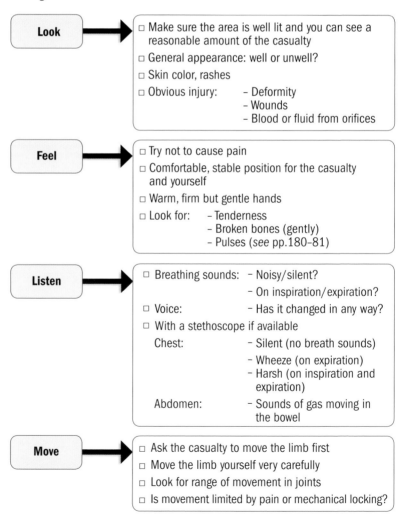

Look
- Make sure the area is well lit and you can see a reasonable amount of the casualty
- General appearance: well or unwell?
- Skin color, rashes
- Obvious injury:
  - Deformity
  - Wounds
  - Blood or fluid from orifices

Feel
- Try not to cause pain
- Comfortable, stable position for the casualty and yourself
- Warm, firm but gentle hands
- Look for:
  - Tenderness
  - Broken bones (gently)
  - Pulses (see pp.180–81)

Listen
- Breathing sounds:
  - Noisy/silent?
  - On inspiration/expiration?
- Voice:
  - Has it changed in any way?
- With a stethoscope if available
  - Chest:
    - Silent (no breath sounds)
    - Wheeze (on expiration)
    - Harsh (on inspiration and expiration)
  - Abdomen:
    - Sounds of gas moving in the bowel

Move
- Ask the casualty to move the limb first
- Move the limb yourself very carefully
- Look for range of movement in joints
- Is movement limited by pain or mechanical locking?

Values for the adult body's vital signs

Vital sign	Normal range	Seriously unwell
Pulse (beats/minute)	50–100	<40 or >130
Systolic blood pressure (mmHg)	100–140	<90
Skin blanch test (capillary refill test, see p.181)	<2 secs	>4 secs
Breathing rate (breaths per minute)	10–20	<8 or >25
Temperature	96.8–99.5°F (36–37.5°C)	<95 or >101°F (35–38.3°C)
Urine output (ml/hour)	40–100	<20

Examining body systems

This should be done in a methodical manner, moving through each body system in turn. It is common sense to start investigating the body system that appears to be experiencing the main problem. The only exception to this general rule is when major trauma or collapse has occurred. In these cases, follow the resuscitation and emergency assessment guidelines (see pp.28–33). A guide to examining the body systems, which outlines important symptoms and signs, is included on p.33.

Monitoring

Monitoring starts when the casualty is first assessed and should continue until the casualty is better or has been evacuated. Routine monitoring should be carried out every hour; if the casualty is very unwell, monitoring should be carried out at least every 15 minutes. An example of a monitoring chart for vital signs is provided on pp.216–217.

Testing

There are a number of simple but effective tests that can be performed relatively easily and may contribute significantly to diagnosis and treatment.
□ Blood sugars
□ Urine analysis (dipstick)
□ Pregnancy test
□ Stool color/consistency
□ Sputum color/amount
□ Temperature

Record keeping

It is very important that you keep details of the history and examination as you go along. Facts and figures are very easily forgotten, and the medical record may well be of considerable importance for the support medical team. An example of a medical reporting chart is included on pp.218–219.

RESUSCITATION—ABC

If an expedition member collapses, resuscitation should be carried out immediately. Every second is vitally important. The expedition medic should learn the basic and advanced life support algorithms and rehearse them on a regular basis. Absolute familiarity with resuscitation procedures could make the difference between life and death.

Basic life support

The basic life support (BLS) algorithm is straightfoward and gives you a clear course of action if a team member falls unconscious. First, stabilize the neck (cervical spine) if there is any chance of injury (*see* pp.178-79). The algorithm prioritizes the most immediate threats to life: opening and maintaining an adequate **A**irway, followed by assessment and treatment of **B**reathing, then assessment and treatment of **C**irculation (ABC).

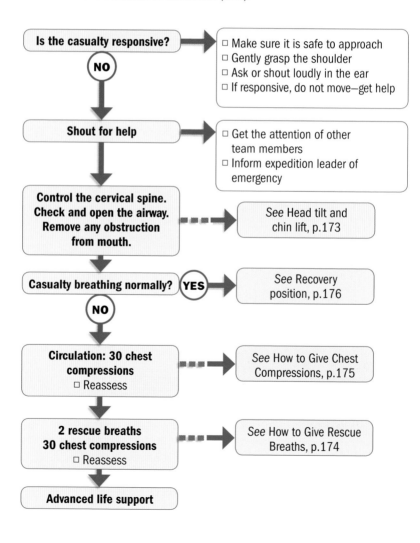

Is the casualty responsive?

NO

- □ Make sure it is safe to approach
- □ Gently grasp the shoulder
- □ Ask or shout loudly in the ear
- □ If responsive, do not move—get help

Shout for help

- □ Get the attention of other team members
- □ Inform expedition leader of emergency

Control the cervical spine. Check and open the airway. Remove any obstruction from mouth.

See Head tilt and chin lift, p.173

Casualty breathing normally? YES

See Recovery position, p.176

NO

Circulation: 30 chest compressions
□ Reassess

See How to Give Chest Compressions, p.175

2 rescue breaths 30 chest compressions
□ Reassess

See How to Give Rescue Breaths, p.174

Advanced life support

Advanced life support

For advanced life support (ALS), you will need an automated external defibrillator (AED) and specific drugs—epinephrine and atropine. The process is more complex than BLS and requires more expertise. If there is any possibility of injury to the spine, stabilize the neck (cervical spine) before you begin (see pp.178–79).

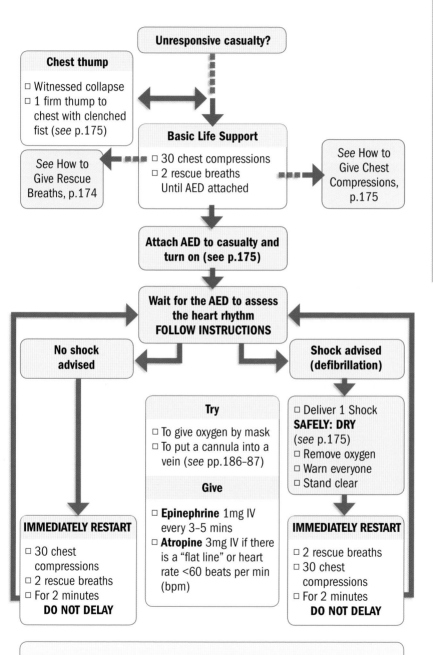

Unresponsive casualty?

Chest thump

- ☐ Witnessed collapse
- ☐ 1 firm thump to chest with clenched fist (see p.175)

See How to Give Rescue Breaths, p.174

Basic Life Support

- ☐ 30 chest compressions
- ☐ 2 rescue breaths
  Until AED attached

See How to Give Chest Compressions, p.175

Attach AED to casualty and turn on (see p.175)

Wait for the AED to assess the heart rhythm FOLLOW INSTRUCTIONS

No shock advised

Shock advised (defibrillation)

Try

- ☐ To give oxygen by mask
- ☐ To put a cannula into a vein (see pp.186–87)

Give

- ☐ **Epinephrine** 1mg IV every 3–5 mins
- ☐ **Atropine** 3mg IV if there is a "flat line" or heart rate <60 beats per min (bpm)

☐ Deliver 1 Shock
SAFELY: DRY (see p.175)
- ☐ Remove oxygen
- ☐ Warn everyone
- ☐ Stand clear

IMMEDIATELY RESTART

- ☐ 30 chest compressions
- ☐ 2 rescue breaths
- ☐ For 2 minutes
  DO NOT DELAY

IMMEDIATELY RESTART

- ☐ 2 rescue breaths
- ☐ 30 chest compressions
- ☐ For 2 minutes
  DO NOT DELAY

Continue until the casualty is breathing, medical help arrives or you are exhausted and cannot continue

ASSESSMENT OF A SICK OR INJURED CASUALTY

Assessment of a very sick or injured casualty must be carried out as quickly as possible. In some cases, several issues will need attention. The system of primary and secondary survey will help you to prioritize your tasks. Practice the surveys as you would practice resuscitation guidelines—until they become second nature.

The framework prioritizes the most immediate threats to life. Deal with each stage effectively before you move on; this is vital. If the Airway, is blocked, an unconscious team member will not live long. Only once the Airway is secure should you then assess Breathing, Circulation and so on. Make sure you are not placing yourself in the path of danger during the assessment.

THE PRIMARY SURVEY

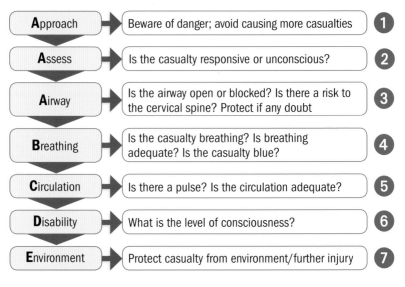

Approach ➡ Beware of danger; avoid causing more casualties ①

Assess ➡ Is the casualty responsive or unconscious? ②

Airway ➡ Is the airway open or blocked? Is there a risk to the cervical spine? Protect if any doubt ③

Breathing ➡ Is the casualty breathing? Is breathing adequate? Is the casualty blue? ④

Circulation ➡ Is there a pulse? Is the circulation adequate? ⑤

Disability ➡ What is the level of consciousness? ⑥

Environment ➡ Protect casualty from environment/further injury ⑦

① Avoid self-injury while approaching casualty

- ☐ Clear obstacles
- ☐ Avoid hazards: e.g. cliff edges
- ☐ Wear protective equipment
- ☐ Beware of live electrical sources

② Assessment: responsive or unconscious?

Assess	Action
☐ Speak loudly in casualty's ear ☐ Grasp the shoulder firmly ☐ Response is normal if breathing and circulation are adequate	☐ If response is normal, make casualty comfortable and go to secondary survey ☐ If response is abnormal, complete primary survey

3 Protection of airway and cervical spine

Assess	Action
□ Unconscious or distressed? □ Seesaw breathing (chest/ abdomen moving in opposite directions)? □ Noisy breathing? □ Effort on inspiration? □ Injury to mouth/face/neck?	□ Stabilize the cervical spine if there is history of injury to head or neck (see pp.178–79) □ Open airway using "head tilt/chin lift" method (see p.173) □ Check mouth/throat for obstructing objects □ Use airway device if available (see pp.173–74)

4 Breathing

Assess	Action
□ Blue or pale? □ Chest moving up and down? □ Rapid, shallow breathing? □ Measure rate of breathing	□ Start BLS if not breathing □ Give oxygen if breathing □ Put in the recovery position if this helps □ Treat pneumothorax if possible (see p.194)

5 Circulation and control of bleeding

Assess	Action
□ Confused or anxious? □ Cold, sweaty face, hands, feet? □ Obvious bleeding? □ Measure pulse rate, blood pressure, and capillary refill	□ Start BLS if no pulse □ Lie flat and raise legs □ Control bleeding (see p.90) □ Insert a cannula into a vein (see pp.186–87) □ Give IV fluids (see pp.188–89) □ Keep warm

6 Disability

Assess	Action

□ Level of consciousness
  A - **A**lert
  V - responds to **V**oice
  P - responds to **P**ain
  U - **U**nresponsive
□ Are the pupils equal and
responding to light?
	□ If conscious level is reduced but casualty is
	breathing: place in recovery position
	□ Continue to treat any other problems
	□ Reassess frequently
	□ Keep warm

7 Environment: protect casualty

Assess	Action
□ Increasingly cool and mottled skin □ Shivering □ Low temperature	□ Keep exposure time to a minimum □ Remove casualty from the exposed position as soon as possible □ Keep warm and dry

THE SECONDARY SURVEY

The secondary survey is a comprehensive, head-to-toe evaluation, which includes both a complete history and a thorough examination. This system is designed to ensure that no serious medical issues or injuries are overlooked. A **"distracting injury,"** such as a compound ("open") fracture of the femur, may divert attention from broken ribs, which may only be discovered days later, unless the whole body is examined carefully.

The history should include two elements: the casualty's previous medical history, and an accurate report of the events leading up to the accident. If the casualty is unconscious, the history may come from others, such as friends and people who witnessed the accident.

Remember that any threats to life must be dealt with in the primary survey, which may take considerable time, before the secondary survey can begin.

Approach the examination with sensitivity. The examination can be confined to the ankle if only the ankle is injured, but should be comprehensive. You may need to undress the casualty to expose either part of or the whole body. Try to respect the dignity and privacy of the casualty while you are doing this, though expediency is the priority.

The history

AMPLE is a simple memory aid that covers all the vital elements of the history.

Allergies ▶ Common, especially reactions to some antibiotics, and can threaten life, making a bad situation worse.

Medication ▶ What does the casualty usually take? Some medications may cause side effects and confuse the situation.

Past Illnesses ▶ Ongoing medical complaints such as diabetes may have significant impact on the current situation. A list of any current medications often helps to identify past illnesses.

Last meal ▶ Time of the last meal will indicate whether the stomach is likely to be full. A full stomach increases the chance of vomiting, especially if unconscious.

Events ▶ Knowing what happened and when will help you to anticipate the nature and severity of injuries. A fall from a height will probably lead to more serious injuries than falling over on the ground. Try to establish:

- **What** happened?
- **Where** did it happen?
- **When** did it happen?
- **How** did it happen?
- **Why** did it happen? (for future prevention)

The examination

Carry out as thorough an examination as possible, within the limits imposed by circumstance. You won't be able to complete a thorough examination in the middle of the night or during bad weather, but you must keep careful notes of any aspects of the examination still to be completed.

The basis for any examination is: **Look, Feel, Listen, Move.** You won't need to undress and examine the whole body if somebody has stubbed their toe, but you **must evaluate from head to toe** if the casualty has fallen down a cliff and been recovered unconscious. Use your common sense, but be more meticulous if there is any uncertainty. Check the front, back and both sides of the body; the examination is not complete until the casualty has been log-rolled onto their side so that the back and spine can be examined (see p.177). Check for medic alert bracelets, necklaces and operation scars before you start, and look inside the pockets for any medications the casualty may be taking.

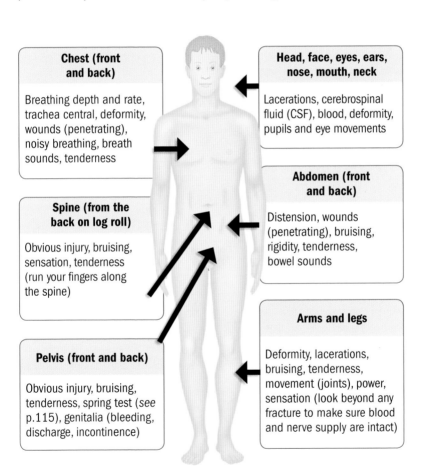

Chest (front and back)

Breathing depth and rate, trachea central, deformity, wounds (penetrating), noisy breathing, breath sounds, tenderness

Head, face, eyes, ears, nose, mouth, neck

Lacerations, cerebrospinal fluid (CSF), blood, deformity, pupils and eye movements

Abdomen (front and back)

Distension, wounds (penetrating), bruising, rigidity, tenderness, bowel sounds

Spine (from the back on log roll)

Obvious injury, bruising, sensation, tenderness (run your fingers along the spine)

Arms and legs

Deformity, lacerations, bruising, tenderness, movement (joints), power, sensation (look beyond any fracture to make sure blood and nerve supply are intact)

Pelvis (front and back)

Obvious injury, bruising, tenderness, spring test (see p.115), genitalia (bleeding, discharge, incontinence)

Remember: continue to monitor for deterioration

MANAGING THE UNCONSCIOUS CASUALTY

An unconscious casualty, perhaps sick or injured, may need to be cared for until help arrives or evacuation can be arranged. You may know why the casualty is unconscious (if an accident has caused a head injury, for example), but some cases may require further examination and testing that is impossible in a wilderness setting. There are several support tasks that the medic, leader and expedition members will need to carry out until medical help is available.

An unconscious casualty is dependent and vulnerable. The goal of the entire team is to sustain the casualty and make sure he reaches safety and medical help in the shortest possible time and in the best possible condition. Aim to avoid deterioration, thereby improving the casualty's chances of recovery.

Maintenance of the airway

An unconscious casualty will not be able to maintain an airway lying on his back.
□ Place the casualty in the recovery position (*see* p.176) as soon as possible.
□ Use airway devices if necessary (*see* pp.173–74).
□ Monitor the following at all times:
  – Change in color
  – Noisy breathing
  – Chest movement
  – Rate of breathing

Recovery position

Place the unconscious casualty in the recovery position (*see* p.176) to maintain the airway and ensure that fluids, such as vomit and saliva, drain out of the mouth and not down the airway into the lungs.
□ Use the "log roll" in possible spinal injury (particularly neck injury, *see* p.177).
□ Keep arms and legs straight if they are injured or fractured.
□ Place the casualty in a safe and secure position, with no risk of further injury.

Injuries

□ Splint/immobilize all fractures if possible.
□ Control bleeding, then clean wounds carefully and dress with a sterile dressing.
□ Review injuries every few hours if evacuation is delayed.

Warmth

□ Make sure the casualty is warm and dry.
□ Monitor the temperature with a thermometer under the armpit.

Pain relief

□ Despite being unconscious, the casualty may still feel pain, which will be particularly severe if he or she is moved.
□ Look for signs of pain (see p.129).
□ Use pain relief carefully:
  – Try not to give opiates (morphine) to head-injured patients
  – If you do use opiates, monitor the rate and depth of respiration
□ Use nonsedating painkillers (such as diclofenac suppositories).
□ Use nerve blocks where possible (see p.199).
□ Immobilize fractures and attempt to reduce the broken ends (see pp.206–207).

Pressure areas and sores

□ If left in the same position for several hours, an immobile casualty will start to develop pressure sores on their skin. Pressure sores may also start to develop underneath padded or inflatable splints.
□ Injuries, cold, incontinence, dehydration and low blood pressure will exacerbate pressure sores.
□ If other injuries allow, you may need to log roll the casualty from side to side every few hours.
□ If the casualty has been secured on a rigid spinal board, take them off, carefully, as soon as possible.

Urinary catheter and nasogastric tube

□ Insert a urinary catheter (see p.201) if evacuation is going to take longer than a few hours—a full bladder will cause a lot of pain.
□ If there is blood at the end of the penis or coming out of the vagina, take extra care over inserting any tubes.
□ A nasogastric tube (see p.200) is useful for two reasons:
  – It can be used to decompress the stomach, reducing the risk of vomiting
  – It can be used as a route to hydrate the casualty.
□ Do not insert a nasogastric tube if there is a possibility of head injury. Insert the tube through the mouth into the stomach instead.

Hydration

It is vital that the casualty receives enough fluid while unconscious, but it is difficult to know how much fluid to give. In general terms, a person weighing 70kg will need 3L a day. You may need to give more fluid if:
□ External or internal injuries cause blood loss
□ A hot climate causes heavy sweating
□ Burn injuries are present (see pp.52–53)
□ Blood pressure is low: low blood pressure may be increased by giving additional fluid in 250ml amounts intravenously.
There are various ways of administering fluid and judging the adequacy of hydration (see pp.184–185).

Simple tests in remote areas

These are simple tests that will provide useful information.
- Blood sugar with testing sticks (essential in diabetics)
- Urine with testing sticks (for blood, sugar, signs of kidney or bladder damage)
- Pregnancy testing kit
- Oximetry (high altitude)

Monitoring vital signs

Monitoring will allow you to spot and correct any deterioration in the casualty's condition early. Using a record chart (*see* pp.216–17), note down the following values every hour as a minimum:
- Pulse
- Blood pressure
- Respiratory rate
- Oxygen saturation (if oximeter is available)
- Urine output (if possible)
- Temperature
- Pupil reactions
- Conscious state AVPU: Alert; Vocal stimuli provoke response; Painful stimuli provoke response; Unresponsive (*see* p.182)/Glasgow Coma Score (*see* p.183).

Communication and evacuation

- Seek medical advice early.
- Communicate effectively: prioritize information.
- Identify the person you are speaking with.
- Evacuate at the first opportunity.
- Do not minimize the seriousness of the situation to rescue authorities.
- Make sure you know how to evacuate a casualty (*see* pp.210–11).
- Make sure documentation goes with the casualty.

LOSS OF CONSCIOUSNESS

Some causes of loss of consciousness (LoC) are obvious, others more difficult to identify. The immediate treatment priorities are airway, breathing and circulation (ABC). The casualty is often not completely unconscious but somewhat responsive. If a casualty's level of consciousness reduces to the point that they are unresponsive, this is a very serious situation.

The Glasgow Coma Scale (GCS) (see p.183) measures the consciousness level. It enables you to detect and monitor both improvement and deterioration. The AVPU method (Alert; Vocal stimuli provoke response; Painful stimuli provoke response; Unresponsive) is more straightforward and allows rapid assessment.

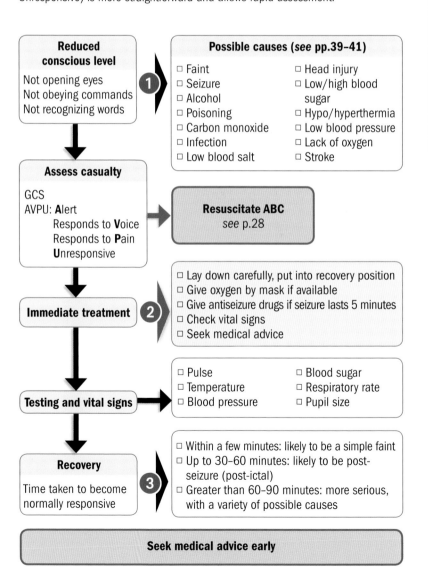

Reduced conscious level

Not opening eyes
Not obeying commands
Not recognizing words

①

Possible causes (see pp.39–41)

- Faint
- Seizure
- Alcohol
- Poisoning
- Carbon monoxide
- Infection
- Low blood salt
- Head injury
- Low/high blood sugar
- Hypo/hyperthermia
- Low blood pressure
- Lack of oxygen
- Stroke

Assess casualty

GCS
AVPU: **A**lert
        Responds to **V**oice
        Responds to **P**ain
        Unresponsive

Resuscitate ABC
see p.28

Immediate treatment

②

- Lay down carefully, put into recovery position
- Give oxygen by mask if available
- Give antiseizure drugs if seizure lasts 5 minutes
- Check vital signs
- Seek medical advice

Testing and vital signs

- Pulse
- Temperature
- Blood pressure
- Blood sugar
- Respiratory rate
- Pupil size

Recovery

Time taken to become normally responsive

③

- Within a few minutes: likely to be a simple faint
- Up to 30–60 minutes: likely to be post-seizure (post-ictal)
- Greater than 60–90 minutes: more serious, with a variety of possible causes

Seek medical advice early

❶ Assessing the casualty

A swift examination will uncover details that may allow you to make a diagnosis. Check for:

☐ Vital signs (pulse, blood pressure)
☐ Obvious seizure
☐ Pupil size
☐ Smell of alcohol, ketones (sweet breath)
☐ Paralysis of one side of the face or body

☐ Head injury
☐ Any other injury and bleeding
☐ Rolling eye movements
☐ Tongue biting
☐ Incontinence of urine or feces.

When ascertaining the level of consciousness, use a gradual increase in stimulation to get the casualty to respond. First, ask for a verbal response ("Are you okay?") in a loud voice. If there is no response, grip the shoulder and shake it gently (beware of possible neck injury). If they still don't respond, try one of the following painful stimuli:

☐ Rub the edge of the eye socket under the eyebrow
☐ Rub the center of the chest firmly
☐ Press a pen onto the base of a finger nail.

To make sure the stimulus is reasonable without causing lasting pain or harm, test the stimulus on yourself first.

❷ Treatment of prolonged seizures

If a seizure or series of seizures lasts longer than 5–10 minutes and the casualty does not regain consciousness, administer treatment to avoid permanent brain damage. An episode of seizures lasting longer than 30 minutes is known as *status epilepticus*. This is a grave emergency that may result in permanent brain damage or death.

First line treatment—ABC and oxygen followed by:

☐ Diazepam 10mg
    – Use the injection form rather than the suppository—absorption is faster
    – Repeat at 15-minute intervals up to 40mg (for a person weighing 70kg)

OR

☐ Lorazepam 2–4mg intravenously
    – Repeat once after 20 minutes
    – Lasts for up to 12 hours

Take note: both diazepam and lorazepam have similar actions, and you should not use them together unless you are directed to do so by a doctor. These drugs will cause sedation, reduce the conscious level and may stop respiration, so use them carefully. Flumazenil can counteract these effects, but should also only be used under medical direction.

❸ Recovery of consciousness

The amount of time it takes for the casualty to recover consciousness can help with making a diagnosis. These time frames are only approximate, however, and should not rule out another diagnosis.

In the post-ictal period, the seizure has ended, but the patient has not regained consciousness. This phase usually lasts less than 30 minutes, but may take several hours. The post-ictal period tends to be longer with more prolonged, generalized seizures and when more medication has been given to terminate the seizure.

Causes of loss of consciousness (LoC)

Fainting

Simple fainting is fairly common. It often happens when blood pressure drops temporarily, causing a "blackout." Severe pain, panic attacks, emotional or physical shock (such as the sight of blood) and excessive heat can all bring on a faint. If the casualty twitches while they are unconscious, it is not necessarily an indication of epilepsy. Put the casualty in the recovery position to help restore the blood flow to the brain. The casualty should recover in a few minutes. If the casualty fell when they fainted, examine for injuries.

Seizures

There are many possible causes of seizures:

- Epilepsy
- Alcohol withdrawal
- Recreational drug withdrawal
- Strokes
- Low blood salt (hyponatremia)
- Head injury
- Low blood sugar
- Infection
- Hyperthermia (fever in children)
- Post-diving.

Seizures may be generalized, causing the whole body to shake, or partial, involving only part of the body (such as the eyes or a single muscle group). Partial seizures may be difficult to recognize, but should be dealt with in the same way. People with epilepsy that is well-controlled may be put at risk of seizures by diarrhea and vomiting (which can reduce absorption of anti-epilepsy tablets), work stress, poor nutrition and dehydration. Epileptics might experience a feeling that they are going to have a seizure, which is known as an "aura." If this happens, they must be moved to a safe place before the seizure begins. The first priority is always resuscitation. After resuscitation, administer treatment to stop seizures that last longer than 5 minutes. Check vital signs. The blood sugar level in particular is essential and may guide immediate treatment.

Alcohol

Alchohol often makes people difficult to wake, but this shouldn't be the case in the wilderness. Excessive alchohol consumption may cause seizures and abstention in heavy drinkers can also cause seizures. If alcohol withdrawal is responsible for seizures, it will usually be after 2–3 days without alcohol. A history of recent heavy drinking and breath that smells of alcohol may both indicate a diagnosis of withdrawl. In alcohol-related seizures, there is a risk of vomiting and vomit may enter the lungs while the casualty is unconscious. Put the casualty in the recovery position. Treat and monitor any seizures that last longer than 5 minutes (*see* p.38).

Poisoning

Poisoning that causes a casualty to lose consciousness, whether accidental or deliberate, is a threat to life. Possible causes include prescription drugs such as antidepressants, sedatives and heart treatment drugs, which can also cause seizures, so keep such drugs safe. Poisoning by gas in a vehicle or on a boat is a real risk. If you rescue a victim of gas poisoning, ensure that you are not overcome yourself (*see* p.170 for specific treatments).

Carbon monoxide (CO)

If you use a gas stove or heater in a tent, shelter or hut that is not adequately ventilated, there is a risk of carbon monoxide poisoning. Symptoms may be indistinct, but include nausea, vomiting, headache, confusion, chest pain and, in extreme cases, loss of consciousness. The casualty may look very red in the face—a color that is often described as "cherry red." Investigate the possibility of carbon monoxide poisoning if a group of team members suffer from similar symptoms. Move the casualty away from the source of CO and give them as much oxygen as possible if oxygen is available (see p.170).

Infection

Both meningitis, which is an infection of the membrane covering the brain, and encephalitis (infection of the brain itself) can cause loss of consciousness and seizures. If the casualty has felt increasingly unwell for hours or days beforehand, been running a high temperature and perhaps had a nonblanching rash, infection is more likely. Treat any seizures and give antibiotics at high dosage as soon as possible via IV route (see pp.158–61 for further treatment).

Low blood salt

An insufficient level of sodium in the blood causes a condition known as hyponatremia. Consider this diagnosis in warm, humid conditions if the casualty has been exerting themselves physically and rehydrating with plain water rather than rehydration salts. Prevention is essential, so ensure adequate, appropriate fluid intake for all members of the team. It is impossible to make a firm diagnosis of hyponatremia in the wilderness, so any treatment will be based on suspicion only. The only course of action after carrying out appropriate resuscitation (see pp.28–29) is to give rectal rehydration fluid or IV saline solution (see pp.184–85).

Head injury

Head injury that causes LoC may have also caused injuries to the spine, particularly the neck (cervical spine). Consider the possibility of spinal injury and protect the cervical spine at all times. A GCS of 13 or more indicates mild injury, while a GCS of 8 or less indicates severe injury. The longer the period of LoC, the more severe the injury, and a period of LoC longer than 5 minutes should be treated as significant. Treatment will involve resuscitation and management of the unconscious casualty (see pp.34–35). Closely monitor any casualty who has suffered LoC as a result of head injury for at least 24 hours—they may deteriorate (see p.94 for further treatment).

Low/high blood sugar

Diabetes is often the cause of high or low blood sugar but there are other causes as well. Both conditions, particularly low blood sugar, may lead to seizures or LoC. If any member of your team loses consciousness it is important to check the blood sugar level as soon as possible (see p.51 for further treatment). In known diabetics, a blood sugar check is absolutely crucial.

Hypo/hyperthermia

Hyperthermia is more likely to cause seizures and LoC if the casualty has a core body core temperature above 104°F (40°C). In hypothermia, LoC might occur if the core temperature is below 90°F (32°C). First, treat the seizure, then reverse the hypo- or hyperthermia (for hypothermia *see* pp.62–65 and for hyperthermia *see* pp.66–69).

Low blood pressure

If systolic blood pressure is lower than 70mmHg, the conscious level will probably be reduced. Some team members, particularly those with previous high blood pressure or diabetes may be susceptible to low blood pressure. The fastest way to counteract low blood pressure is to lie the casualty down and raise the legs, restoring blood flow to the head. Next, gain IV access and start fluid resuscitation (*see* pp.184–85). Look for a cause of low blood pressure, such as heart attack or blood loss. The casualty's state may worsen rapidly, so seek medical advice urgently.

Lack of oxygen

Obstruction of the airway, restricted breathing or lack of adequate circulation (as above) can all compromise oxygen delivery to the brain. In addition, oxygen levels can fall dangerously low if open fires or cooking stoves are used in poorly ventilated huts or snow holes. LoC and seizures caused by oxygen shortage are grave and very likely to cause permanent damage. Resuscitate immediately (*see* p.28), and give oxygen by mask if possible. Seizures that last longer than 5 minutes should be treated.

Stroke

When a blood clot or bleed obstructs blood flow to part of the brain, a stroke occurs. A very large stroke or a smaller stroke in a critical area of the brain will cause LoC. Other symptoms include seizures, paralysis or abnormal movements down one side of the body. Resuscitate immediately in order to improve the supply of blood and oxygen to the brain and limit further damage (*see* p.133 for further treatment).

Post-diving

If a diver surfaces and then loses consciousness soon afterward, he or she is likely to have suffered an air embolism. Resuscitation must be carried out immediately. If the casualty is breathing and has a pulse, put them in the recovery position. Give oxygen and administer IV fluids if possible. **Seek urgent medical advice**—aim to evacuate immediately, ideally to a decompression facility.

CHOKING

A team member with a blocked airway who is having difficulty breathing may collapse. Take immediate steps to identify the cause and remove the blockage.

The most common cause is a piece of food stuck in the throat (pharynx), voice box (larynx) or further down, in the wind pipe (trachea). This may also provoke spasm of the muscles of the airway (bronchospasm) or the vocal cords (laryngospasm), exacerbating the blockage of the airway.

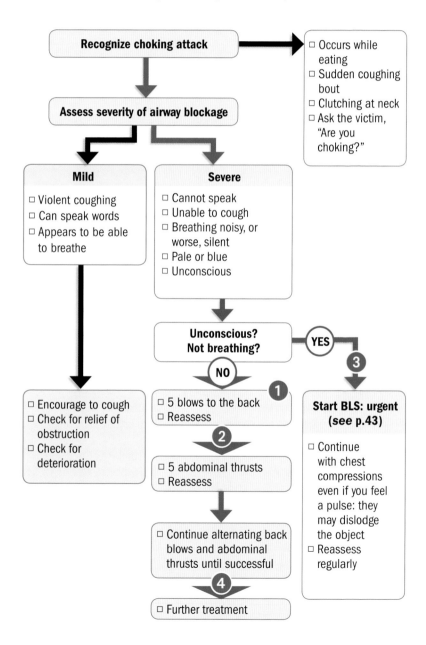

Recognize choking attack

- □ Occurs while eating
- □ Sudden coughing bout
- □ Clutching at neck
- □ Ask the victim, "Are you choking?"

Assess severity of airway blockage

Mild
- □ Violent coughing
- □ Can speak words
- □ Appears to be able to breathe

Severe
- □ Cannot speak
- □ Unable to cough
- □ Breathing noisy, or worse, silent
- □ Pale or blue
- □ Unconscious

Unconscious? Not breathing?

YES → **3**

NO

- □ Encourage to cough
- □ Check for relief of obstruction
- □ Check for deterioration

1
- □ 5 blows to the back
- □ Reassess

2
- □ 5 abdominal thrusts
- □ Reassess

□ Continue alternating back blows and abdominal thrusts until successful

4

□ Further treatment

3
Start BLS: urgent (see p.43)

- □ Continue with chest compressions even if you feel a pulse: they may dislodge the object
- □ Reassess regularly

① Giving back blows

In order for you to do this, the victim must be conscious and standing up. Back blows might cause the victim pain, so describe what you are going to do.

☐ Stand to one side. Lean the victim's upper body well forward over your left arm, supporting the chest. In this position, any dislodged object is more likely to be expelled from the victim's mouth.

☐ Give five sharp and very firm blows between the shoulder blades with the heel of your hand.

☐ Between each blow, reassess; stop delivering blows if the object is dislodged or comes out.

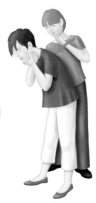

Give five firm blows between the shoulder blades.

② Giving abdominal thrusts

For this procedure also, the victim must be conscious and standing. Describe the procedure to the victim. Abdominal thrusts may cause more pain than back blows.

☐ Stand behind the victim and lean them forward. Place a clenched fist in the upper abdomen, just below the ribs in the center line. Place your other hand over the fist and maintain a firm hold.

☐ Apply up to five sharp thrusts to the abdomen.

☐ Reassess briefly between thrusts, and stop if the object is dislodged or comes out.

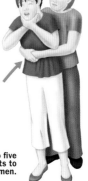

Give up to five sharp thrusts to the abdomen.

③ Basic life support with chest compressions

If the choking victim loses consciousness, you will need to administer basic life support. It is probably worthwhile continuing chest compressions even if you can feel a pulse—the compressions may increase pressure in the lungs to the extent that the object is forced out of the airway. Continue administering compressions until one of the following occurs:

☐ The object is dislodged
☐ There is a pulse
☐ Help arrives
☐ You become exhausted and are unable continue.

④ Further treatment

The victim may remain wheezy, with persistent breathing difficulties, after the object has been dislodged. See pp.172–173 for further supportive treatment.

HEMORRHAGE AND SHOCK

A team member who is injured and bleeding is one of the most alarming emergencies in the wilderness. If the bleeding (hemorrhage) is not stopped rapidly, the casualty may go into shock—when direct medical help is not on hand, shock is a life-threatening condition.

Shock occurs when the body's vital organs are not receiving sufficient blood. Act immediately—there must not be any delay. If bleeding is external, the cause will probably be obvious. If bleeding is internal, the cause will be more difficult to recognize, assess and stop. Injuries that may cause internal bleeding include penetrating injury to chest or abdomen; arm and leg bone fractures; pelvic fractures; and blunt trauma to chest or abdomen. The stomach, intestines, and uterus are other common locations of internal bleeding. The symptoms of shock are listed below and will depend on the amount of blood lost.

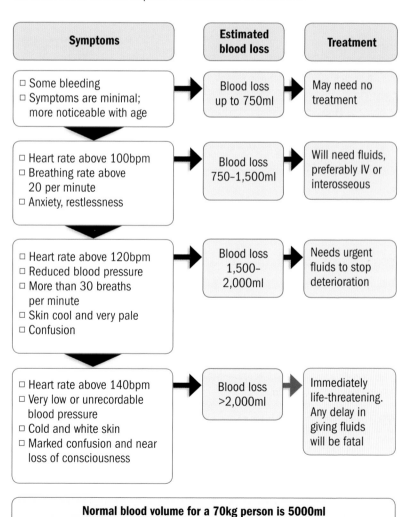

Symptoms	Estimated blood loss	Treatment
□ Some bleeding □ Symptoms are minimal; more noticeable with age	Blood loss up to 750ml	May need no treatment
□ Heart rate above 100bpm □ Breathing rate above 20 per minute □ Anxiety, restlessness	Blood loss 750–1,500ml	Will need fluids, preferably IV or interosseous
□ Heart rate above 120bpm □ Reduced blood pressure □ More than 30 breaths per minute □ Skin cool and very pale □ Confusion	Blood loss 1,500–2,000ml	Needs urgent fluids to stop deterioration
□ Heart rate above 140bpm □ Very low or unrecordable blood pressure □ Cold and white skin □ Marked confusion and near loss of consciousness	Blood loss >2,000ml	Immediately life-threatening. Any delay in giving fluids will be fatal

Normal blood volume for a 70kg person is 5000ml

Immediate treatment

□ Resuscitate ABCDE (*see* pp.28–31).
□ Lie the casualty down and raise the legs.
□ Get IV or intraosseus access if you can and give fluid (*see* p.186 and 188).

How to stop bleeding

Direct pressure
□ Wearing gloves, apply very firm pressure.
□ Press on either side if there are bones sticking out.
□ Continue for as long as possible or until the bleeding stops.

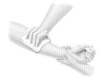

Apply direct pressure.

Splinting
Put the broken ends of the bones back as close as possible to the normal position. Splint firmly (not too tightly) in position. If the pelvis is fractured, hold it together with a strap or sling.

Tie a tourniquet.

Immobilization
Keeping the casualty still gives any clot that forms the best chance of staying in place and sealing up the bleeding point.

Elevation
Elevating the injured part of the body, usually an arm or leg, will reduce bleeding from veins and skin, but is unlikely to be effective with arterial bleeding.

Stitching
Stitching or stapling the wound edges back together may stop bleeding.

Forceps/clamp
Use a clamp or a pair of forceps to pinch off the bleeding point, particularly for spurting (arterial) bleeding.

Tourniquet
Use in extreme circumstances only, as this procedure may dangerously reduce blood flow to distal arm or leg. Tourniquets are essential to stop major hemorrhage following traumatic limb amputation.

Young and older casualties
Younger people can tolerate blood loss to a much greater extent than older people, so treat older people as a priority. However, when young people start to show symptoms of blood loss, their condition is serious and requires urgent treatment.

Blood loss in fractures
□ Fractured humerus, up to 500ml
□ Fractured femur, over 1,000ml per leg
□ Fractured pelvis, 2,000ml or more

Medications that may complicate blood loss
□ Blood-thinning drugs such as aspirin and warfarin are often prescribed for heart conditions. They will exacerbate bleeding and should be stopped.
□ Beta blockers, such as atenolol, slow the heart rate and may hide or suppress the rapid-pulse response to significant blood loss.
□ Anti-motion sickness tablets sometimes cause drowsiness, which exacerbates reduced conscious level caused by severe blood loss.

HEART ATTACK

The heart is essentially a muscle and needs a constant blood supply to keep functioning. The condition called angina occurs when the blood supply is reduced. If the reduction becomes critical, this may cause a heart attack (myocardial infarction), which is usually extremely painful. If a heart attack causes the casualty's heartbeat to become irregular, they may then suffer a fall in blood pressure or even cardiac arrest.

People who are young and fit have heart attacks very rarely. They become more likely with age, especially in people who have previously suffered from angina or had heart attacks in the past. People with a history of heart problems should not take part in long, stressful expeditions. Chest pain has many possible causes, so if a team member becomes symptomatic, evaluate thoroughly.

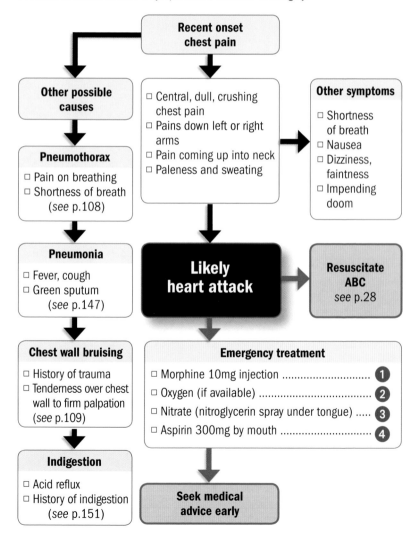

Recent onset chest pain

Other possible causes

Pneumothorax
- Pain on breathing
- Shortness of breath
  (see p.108)

Pneumonia
- Fever, cough
- Green sputum
  (see p.147)

Chest wall bruising
- History of trauma
- Tenderness over chest wall to firm palpation
  (see p.109)

Indigestion
- Acid reflux
- History of indigestion
  (see p.151)

- Central, dull, crushing chest pain
- Pains down left or right arms
- Pain coming up into neck
- Paleness and sweating

Other symptoms
- Shortness of breath
- Nausea
- Dizziness, faintness
- Impending doom

Likely heart attack

Resuscitate ABC
see p.28

Emergency treatment
- Morphine 10mg injection .... ①
- Oxygen (if available) .... ②
- Nitrate (nitroglycerin spray under tongue) ..... ③
- Aspirin 300mg by mouth .... ④

Seek medical advice early

TREATMENT OF HEART ATTACKS

In the event of collapse, immediate resuscitation and advanced life support are essential. Loss of consciousness may be caused by an irregular heart rhythm (ventricular fibrillation or tachycardia), which stops the heart pumping blood properly. Rapid defibrillation with an AED may return the heart back to normal rhythm. If the heart attack is minor, there are a few simple treatments that may prevent the attack from getting worse or happening again—morphine, oxygen, nitrate spray and aspirin (MONA):

➊ Morphine 10mg intramuscular injection

Give this injection into the shoulder, firmly (see p.189). Give an injection of anti-nausea medicine (cyclizine) as well. This will reduce the levels of pain and anxiety in the casualty and lessen the strain on the heart.

➋ Oxygen by face mask (if available)

Place the mask on the casualty's face as soon as possible, with a flow rate of 5–10L per minute. This will increase the supply of oxygen to the heart, reducing further damage to the heart muscle.

➌ Nitroglycerin spray under the tongue

Give a nitroglycerin spray twice under the tongue as soon as possible. The spray will dilate the arteries supplying the heart, increasing blood supply. If the chest pain does not go away or returns, the treatment can be repeated. However, nitroglycerin spray may lower the blood pressure or cause a headache if overused.

➍ Aspirin 300mg by mouth

Give in the dispersible form if possible; absorption from the stomach will be faster. Aspirin will thin the blood and reduce the chance of a clot in the arteries supplying the heart muscle.

Ongoing treatment

This depends on the physical state of the casualty. It is essential to seek medical advice straight away. If advice is not immediately available, continue treatment as follows until help is reached:
▢ Aspirin 150mg per day (as long as stomach is not upset/bleeding)
▢ Nitroglycerin spray if the chest pain returns
▢ Morphine 5mg injections if the chest pain returns, depending on the conscious state of the casualty.

Team member with known heart problems

Any team member with a history of heart problems should be carefully evaluated before departure (see pp.24–25). A person who complains of chest pain in the absence of physical exertion, or who suffers worsening chest pains and finds routine tasks progressively more difficult, should not leave with the expedition and should seek medical advice immediately.

ALLERGY AND ANAPHYLAXIS

Anaphylaxis, or anaphylactic shock, is a severe allergic reaction that affects the entire body. The mouth and throat may swell, and the casualty may collapse due to low blood pressure and inability to breathe. Team members with a history of anaphylactic reactions are likely to know what triggers them and should always carry a preprepared epinephrine syringe for emergencies. Seafood, nuts, bee and wasp stings, drugs (often penicillin), latex rubber and vaccines are all common triggers.

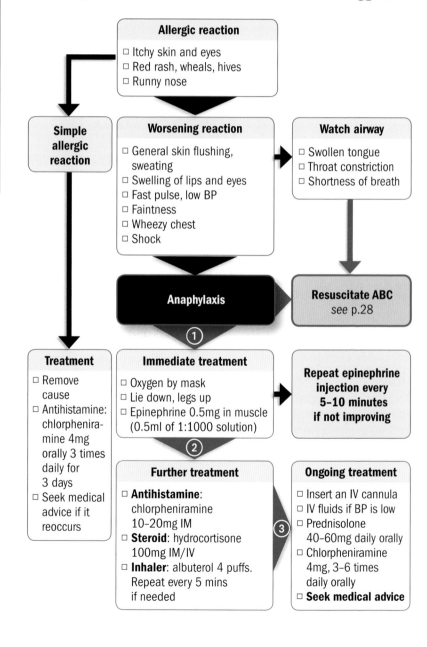

Allergic reaction
- Itchy skin and eyes
- Red rash, wheals, hives
- Runny nose

Simple allergic reaction

Worsening reaction
- General skin flushing, sweating
- Swelling of lips and eyes
- Fast pulse, low BP
- Faintness
- Wheezy chest
- Shock

Watch airway
- Swollen tongue
- Throat constriction
- Shortness of breath

Anaphylaxis

Resuscitate ABC
see p.28

Treatment
- Remove cause
- Antihistamine: chlorphenira-mine 4mg orally 3 times daily for 3 days
- Seek medical advice if it reoccurs

① Immediate treatment
- Oxygen by mask
- Lie down, legs up
- Epinephrine 0.5mg in muscle (0.5ml of 1:1000 solution)

Repeat epinephrine injection every 5–10 minutes if not improving

② Further treatment
- **Antihistamine**: chlorpheniramine 10–20mg IM
- **Steroid**: hydrocortisone 100mg IM/IV
- **Inhaler**: albuterol 4 puffs. Repeat every 5 mins if needed

③ Ongoing treatment
- Insert an IV cannula
- IV fluids if BP is low
- Prednisolone 40–60mg daily orally
- Chlorpheniramine 4mg, 3–6 times daily orally
- **Seek medical advice**

1 Immediate treatment

- ☐ Remove the trigger if possible.
- ☐ Lie the casualty in a comfortable position and raise their legs.
- ☐ Give oxygen by face mask (5L per minute) if available.
- ☐ Epinephrine is the single most important treatment to stop things getting worse.
- ☐ Epinephrine injection 0.5mg (0.5ml of 1:1000 solution) into the front of the thigh or shoulder. This may be repeated every 5-10 minutes if the casualty is not improving. Use a different limb to inject repeat doses.
- ☐ Pre-filled syringes of epinephrine should be used if available.
- ☐ Epinephrine may cause the pulse to go faster, and increase the blood pressure. Be careful the injection doesn't go directly into a blood vessel (*see* p.189).

2 Further treatment

The aim of the following additional treatments is to damp down the anaphylactic reaction more permanently than epinephrine is able to do and to prevent the process from starting up again.

Antihistamine injection:	Chlorpheniramine injection 10-20mg into the front of the thigh or shoulder. Use a different limb to the one used for epinephrine. Give up to 40mg per day. Continue for 24–48 hours post reaction.
Steroid injection:	Hydrocortisone 100mg IM or IV if access available. Begins to work over several hours and has a prolonged effect. Give up to 100mg 3 times per day. Continue for 24–48 hours post reaction.
Inhaler:	Albuterol inhaler 4 puffs, repeated as necessary every 5 minutes. Treats wheeze that may develop with anaphylaxis. Continue for as long as the wheeze is present.

3 Ongoing treatment

The goal here is to stabilize the casualty, prevent the anaphylactic reaction returning, and to secure medical help as soon as possible.

IV fluid:	Fluid resuscitation may be required in the early stages if the blood pressure remains dangerously low despite the other treatments (*see* pp.186-187).
Oral steroids:	Continue oral prednisolone 40-60mg per day according to symptoms.
Oral antihistamines:	Continue oral chlorpheniramine 4mg 3-6 times per day according to symptoms.

> **Continue oral treatment until casualty is under medical care.**
> **Seek medical advice early**

DIABETIC EMERGENCIES

Expedition members may have one of three types of diabetes: diabetes that is controlled by an injection of insulin a few times a day; diabetes controlled with oral diabetic tablets; or diabetes that has not been previously diagnosed (that is, the team member has diabetic problems for the first time).

The blood sugar may be too high (too little insulin, too few tablets or too much food), or too low (too much insulin, too many tablets or too little food). Testing blood sugar levels using testing sticks is simple, and will aid treatment.

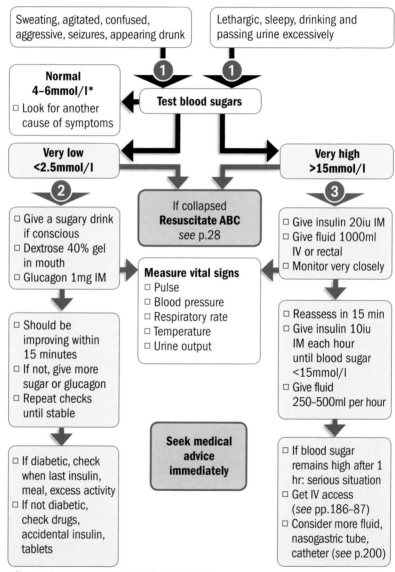

Sweating, agitated, confused, aggressive, seizures, appearing drunk

Lethargic, sleepy, drinking and passing urine excessively

1 **1**

Test blood sugars

**Normal
4–6mmol/l***
□ Look for another cause of symptoms

**Very low
<2.5mmol/l**

**Very high
>15mmol/l**

2

3

If collapsed
Resuscitate ABC
see p.28

□ Give a sugary drink if conscious
□ Dextrose 40% gel in mouth
□ Glucagon 1mg IM

□ Give insulin 20iu IM
□ Give fluid 1000ml IV or rectal
□ Monitor very closely

Measure vital signs
□ Pulse
□ Blood pressure
□ Respiratory rate
□ Temperature
□ Urine output

□ Should be improving within 15 minutes
□ If not, give more sugar or glucagon
□ Repeat checks until stable

□ Reassess in 15 min
□ Give insulin 10iu IM each hour until blood sugar <15mmol/l
□ Give fluid 250–500ml per hour

Seek medical advice immediately

□ If diabetic, check when last insulin, meal, excess activity
□ If not diabetic, check drugs, accidental insulin, tablets

□ If blood sugar remains high after 1 hr: serious situation
□ Get IV access (see pp.186–87)
□ Consider more fluid, nasogastric tube, catheter (see p.200)

* Glucose units: to convert mmol/l to mg/dl, multiply by 18

❶ Testing blood sugar

To test blood sugar, prick a fingertip, squeeze a drop of blood onto the testing stick, wait the amount of time specified in the instructions, then read the result.

❷ Treating low blood sugar

In a known diabetic, low blood sugar may result from excess insulin, too many tablets, lack of food, or strenuous exercise. Some diabetics will be aware that they are having a "hypo," others may simply collapse. It is unusual for people without diabetes to have very low blood sugar—possible causes include drugs, alcohol, malaria or an accidental dose of insulin or tablets.

Giving sugar

If the casualty is conscious, give them a cookie or sweet drink. Concentrated 40% dextrose gel can be placed under the tongue, rubbed into the inside of the cheek or swallowed, but do not put food in the casualty's mouth if he or she is unconscious as it may be aspirated into the lungs.

Glucagon

In unconscious casualties, consider giving 1mg of glucagon intramuscularly (into the shoulder or front of thigh), or intravenously if access is available.

History

If the casualty is a known diabetic, ask when the last dose of insulin or tablet was given and the time of the last meal. Doses may need to be altered. With a casualty who is not a diabetic, find out if this has happened before and any history of drugs or illnesses.

❸ Treating high blood sugar

With a known diabetic, this may be due to too little insulin or too few tablets, or it may mean the casualty is unwell, for instance with an infection. An undiagnosed diabetic who is having problems for the first time will need medical help as soon as possible. If there are testing sticks for urine available, test the urine for sugar and ketones. The medical advisor will want this information. As the casualty improves, the level of sugar and ketones in the urine should reduce.

Insulin

The best way to treat is to give insulin injections intramuscularly into the shoulder or front of thigh. Give 20 units at first, then 10 units per hour until the sugar level starts to fall. Seek medical advice early to guide insulin management.

Fluid

The casualty will probably be very dehydrated. Give 1L of fluid intravenously over the first 30 minutes if you have access to IV fluid. If IV access is not possible, use the rectal route (see p.202) if unconscious. After 30 minutes, lessen the amount of fluid to about 250-500ml per hour. The aim is to keep urine output at about 50-100ml per hour. Seek medical advice early to guide fluid management.

If the sugars remain too high after one hour

Medical advice is absolutely necessary at this time. It is very important to gain IV access and to pass a urinary catheter. Consider putting in a nasogastric (NG) tube to empty the stomach (particularly if the casualty is unconscious); this can be a route for giving fluid. If the casualty has a temperature above 100°F (38°C), give a dose of IV antibiotic. Check allergies first.

BURNS

Any significant burn should be recognized as a major injury affecting the whole body and assessed with primary and secondary surveys to ensure no additional injuries are overlooked (see pp.30–33). The airway may be particularly at risk, especially with fires in enclosed spaces, such as a shelter or tent. The casualty may get worse in the hours after the accident. The aim of treatment is to stop the burning process as quickly as possible, to limit damage. After urgent resuscitation, appropriate fluid replacement is absolutely crucial.

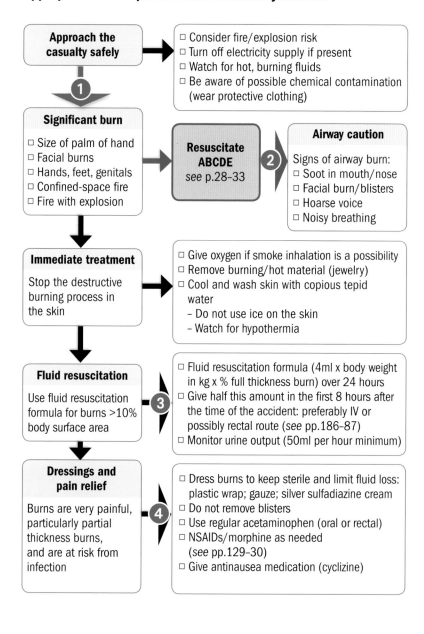

Approach the casualty safely

- ☐ Consider fire/explosion risk
- ☐ Turn off electricity supply if present
- ☐ Watch for hot, burning fluids
- ☐ Be aware of possible chemical contamination (wear protective clothing)

1

Significant burn

- ☐ Size of palm of hand
- ☐ Facial burns
- ☐ Hands, feet, genitals
- ☐ Confined-space fire
- ☐ Fire with explosion

Resuscitate ABCDE see p.28–33

2

Airway caution

Signs of airway burn:
- ☐ Soot in mouth/nose
- ☐ Facial burn/blisters
- ☐ Hoarse voice
- ☐ Noisy breathing

Immediate treatment

Stop the destructive burning process in the skin

- ☐ Give oxygen if smoke inhalation is a possibility
- ☐ Remove burning/hot material (jewelry)
- ☐ Cool and wash skin with copious tepid water
  - Do not use ice on the skin
  - Watch for hypothermia

Fluid resuscitation

Use fluid resuscitation formula for burns >10% body surface area

3

- ☐ Fluid resuscitation formula (4ml x body weight in kg x % full thickness burn) over 24 hours
- ☐ Give half this amount in the first 8 hours after the time of the accident: preferably IV or possibly rectal route (see pp.186–87)
- ☐ Monitor urine output (50ml per hour minimum)

Dressings and pain relief

Burns are very painful, particularly partial thickness burns, and are at risk from infection

4

- ☐ Dress burns to keep sterile and limit fluid loss: plastic wrap; gauze; silver sulfadiazine cream
- ☐ Do not remove blisters
- ☐ Use regular acetaminophen (oral or rectal)
- ☐ NSAIDs/morphine as needed (see pp.129–30)
- ☐ Give antinausea medication (cyclizine)

History

- ☐ Finding out exactly what happened as soon as possible may give some idea as to the severity of the injury.
- ☐ Try to find out exactly how long ago the accident happened (it may be obvious), as this will guide fluid resuscitation.
- ☐ Factors causing more severe burns: prolonged exposure; becoming unconscious for any period; contact with flammables; confined space; explosion.

1 Examination: assessment of burns

Burn area
- ☐ The area of a burn is estimated as a percentage of the body surface area (BSA).
- ☐ The area of full thickness burn should be estimated, as this type causes more fluid loss and more significant complications.
- ☐ Larger burn areas cause more complications.
- ☐ Mildly reddened skin may become obvious full thickness burn over the hours following the accident.
- ☐ Knowing the area of full thickness burn is important, and there are various ways of estimating it.
- ☐ For small burns, the area can be estimated by assuming the area of the casualty's palm is 1% BSA and then mapping the area of burn.
- ☐ For larger burns, there is the "rule of nines." This assumes each region of the body is approximately 9% BSA (see p.54 for body map).

**The area of full thickness burn is frequently underestimated.
Keep monitoring and reassess the type and area of burn.**

Recognizing the type of burn

Superficial burn: Reddened skin, similar to sunburn. Painful and tender to touch.

Partial thickness (PT) burn: Blistered skin, with red, healthy, soft tissue underneath the blisters. Very painful and tender, as all the nerve endings are still intact.

Full thickness (FT) burn: Pale, leathery area, burnt through to the underlying layers. May be charred, involving structures like muscle, tendon, and bone. The burn itself tends not to be painful, as all the nerve endings have been destroyed. However, the area around an FT burn may be extremely painful.

Significant burns
Burns to particular regions of the body are very significant because of longer term complications: face, hands, feet, genitals.

**If significant burns occur,
seek medical advice immediately.**

Rule of Nines

- ☐ Each region of the body (arm, front/back of leg, front/back of chest, front/back of abdomen) counts as 9% BSA.
- ☐ Count obvious FT burns and blistered skin. Exclude reddened skin, but monitor, as these areas may progress to FT burn and will need adding into the total area.

❷ Risks to the airway

Serious burns pose a threat to the airway. If burns do affect the airway, you should seek medical advice immediately. The situation could threaten life as tissue swelling worsens in the hours following the accident.

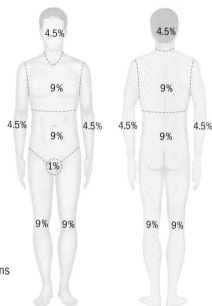

Rule of Nines: body map

Danger signs to look out for:

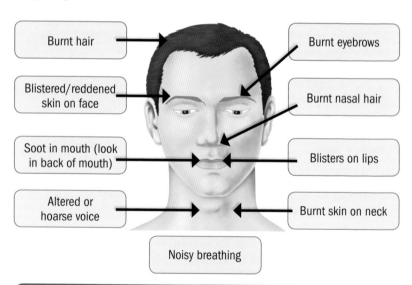

Burnt hair

Burnt eyebrows

Blistered/reddened skin on face

Burnt nasal hair

Soot in mouth (look in back of mouth)

Blisters on lips

Altered or hoarse voice

Burnt skin on neck

Noisy breathing

> **If any of these signs are present, seek medical advice and arrange evacuation immediately**

The outlook is very grave if the casualty does begin to struggle with breathing. The only course of action in the wilderness is to give oxygen if available. The casualty should be kept sitting upright as long as possible to minimize swelling. Attempt resuscitation if the casualty collapses, but resuscitation is unlikely to succeed in these circumstances. Intubation or surgical airway should only be undertaken by trained and experienced medical practitioners. Seek medical advice.

③ Fluid resuscitation

□ Any FT or PT burn over 10% BSA may need fluid resuscitation either intravenously or rectally if unconscious.
□ Get IV access in unburnt part as soon as possible (*see* p.186).

The formula for fluid resuscitation is 4ml x %BSA FT burn x weight (kg)
□ Give half this amount in the first 8 hours following the accident.
□ Give the remaining half over the next 16 hours.
□ Use normal (0.9%) saline fluid or Ringer's lactate solution, given intravenously or rectally, or salt replacement fluid given rectally or orally.
□ This is only a guide and the casualty should be reassessed frequently.

□ Urine output:
  – A minimum 50ml per hour
  – Give a fluid bolus of 250ml if urine output is below this
  – Put in a urinary catheter if necessary (*see* p.186)
□ Fluid resuscitation may have to continue for 36 hours or more.
□ If you are fluid resuscitating, you must seek medical advice, to know what complications may occur and to know when to stop.

④ Cleaning and dressing burns

□ Burns pose the risks of losing fluid from the body and infection. The dressings reduce these risks.
□ Nonadherent material should be removed from the burn area.
□ Chemical burns need washing with copious water ("The solution to pollution is dilution.") Water should be clean but not necessarily drinking standard.
□ Replace dressings every 2–3 days according to the state of the burn.
□ Apply silver sulfadiazine cream to burnt hands and feet and put in plastic bags.
□ Genitals and face can be coated in petroleum jelly and not dressed.
□ Do not remove blisters as they make excellent natural sterile dressings.
□ Elevate affected areas as much as possible to reduce swelling.
□ Use antibiotics if there are signs of infection (*see* inside back cover).

Plastic wrap If nothing else is on hand, take a few winds off a roll of plastic wrap, then use the next part for dressing. Do not wind tightly, just lay it on.
Dressing Use a paraffin-impregnated dressing with a sterile gauze patch over the top to hold it in place.
Silver sulfadiazine A silver sulfadiazine cream can be used to prevent infection and fluid loss. Do not use on the face as it may cause gray coloring of the skin.
Hydrocolloid These dressings protect wounds from contamination, hold in water and can stay in place for a few days. They can be used for awkward areas.
Petroleum jelly To seal wounds and prevent moisture loss, petroleum jelly can be used as an emergency dressing for difficult areas, such as the face and genitals.
Honey If nothing else is available, spread honey on gauze, work it in and then use the pieces of gauze for dressing burns.

HIGH ALTITUDE

Above 3,500m, many travelers experience symptoms of acute mountain sickness (AMS); a few of these progress to high-altitude cerebral edema (HACE) and/or high altitude pulmonary edema (HAPE). In addition, problems caused by extreme cold (see pp.62–65) become more serious at altitude.

Proper acclimatization is the key to avoiding these life-threatening conditions. If they do occur, prompt recognition and knowledge of the effective treatments will save lives. For a guide to diagnosing AMS—the Lake Louise AMS Score—see p.220-221.

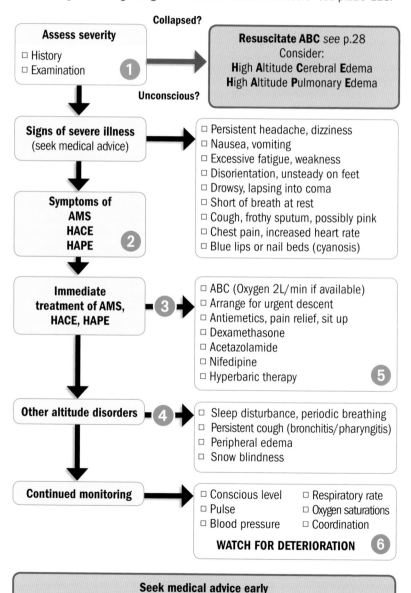

Assess severity
- History
- Examination
1

Collapsed?

Unconscious?

Resuscitate ABC see p.28
Consider:
High **A**ltitude **C**erebral **E**dema
High **A**ltitude **P**ulmonary **E**dema

Signs of severe illness
(seek medical advice)

- Persistent headache, dizziness
- Nausea, vomiting
- Excessive fatigue, weakness
- Disorientation, unsteady on feet
- Drowsy, lapsing into coma
- Short of breath at rest
- Cough, frothy sputum, possibly pink
- Chest pain, increased heart rate
- Blue lips or nail beds (cyanosis)

**Symptoms of
AMS
HACE
HAPE**
2

**Immediate
treatment of AMS,
HACE, HAPE**
3

- ABC (Oxygen 2L/min if available)
- Arrange for urgent descent
- Antiemetics, pain relief, sit up
- Dexamethasone
- Acetazolamide
- Nifedipine
- Hyperbaric therapy
5

Other altitude disorders
4

- Sleep disturbance, periodic breathing
- Persistent cough (bronchitis/pharyngitis)
- Peripheral edema
- Snow blindness

Continued monitoring

- Conscious level
- Pulse
- Blood pressure
- Respiratory rate
- Oxygen saturations
- Coordination

WATCH FOR DETERIORATION
6

Seek medical advice early

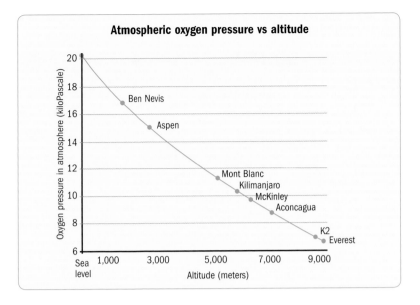

Atmospheric oxygen pressure vs altitude

1 History and examination

- Rapid ascent to altitudes above 2,400m increases the risk of AMS, HACE, and HAPE.
- Absolute altitude is also a factor, with more severe symptoms at higher altitudes.
- A previous history of illness at high altitude increases the risk of repeat problems.

Important points in the history	Important points in the examination
<ul><li>When did the symptoms start?</li><li>Physical performance in comparison with rest of group</li><li>Rate of ascent and rest days</li><li>Altitude when last well</li><li>Previous history of AMS etc.</li><li>Previous history of lung or heart problems</li><li>Recent throat/chest infections</li><li>Normal medications</li></ul>	**Look** <ul><li>Signs of confusion, unsteadiness</li><li>Rate of breathing, distress</li><li>Signs of cyanosis (blue lips and fingers)</li><li>Nature and color of sputum</li></ul>**Listen** Chest for crackles on breathing **Document** Vital signs, treatments, timings, response

2 Onset of symptoms

AMS Onset typically around 6–12 hours after arrival at altitude, usually resolves after 72–96 hours.

HACE Usually (but not always) preceded by AMS that does not resolve after 72–96 hours. Can be sudden in onset. HACE will be exacerbated by difficulties in breathing if HAPE also occurs.

HAPE May develop either very rapidly or over 48–72 hours after arrival at altitude. May occur at anytime while at altitude, even after having descended from greater altitude. HAPE may occur without symptoms of HACE.

Symptoms and signs of AMS, HACE and HAPE

AMS	HACE	HAPE
Symptoms	**Symptoms**	**Symptoms**
	Symptoms of AMS plus:	Symptoms of AMS plus:
☐ Headache, worse when lying down or bending over	☐ Persistent headache not easily relieved by analgesics	☐ Short of breath on minimal exertion or at rest
☐ Dizziness, lightheaded	☐ Confusion, disorientation	☐ Increasingly tired and fatigued
☐ Lack of appetite	☐ Drowsiness	☐ Cough with or without sputum
☐ Increasingly tired and fatigued	☐ Bad coordination when performing simple tasks	☐ Chest pain
☐ Frequent awakening even when tired	☐ Increasingly tired and fatigued	☐ Frequent awakening even when tired
	☐ Blurred or double vision	☐ Other symptoms of HACE
Signs	**Signs**	**Signs**
Little in the way of signs initially, but bad coordination, difficulty walking, confusion, drowsiness **indicate worsening and onset of HACE**.	☐ Reduced consciousness, coma	☐ Increased breathing rate >20/min
Symptoms and signs of HAPE may also be present.	☐ Difficulty with walking (ataxic gait), standing with eyes closed	☐ Increased heart rate >90/min at rest
	☐ Signs of stroke	☐ Temperature about 100–101°F (38–38.5°C)
	☐ Blue lips, fingers, hypoxia on pulse oximeter (see below)	☐ Blue lips, fingers, hypoxia on pulse oximeter (see below)
	☐ Crackles in chest on breathing	☐ Crackles in chest on breathing
	☐ Symptoms and signs of HAPE may also be present	

③ Immediate treatment of AMS, HACE and HAPE

Oxygen Give immediately if available. Use as a "bridge" until descent, hyperbaric therapy etc. have been arranged. Watch reserves: 2L/min from a portable size cylinder (Size D) will last less than 3 hours.

Urgent descent Treat as an emergency. Do not delay to arrange helicopters or other forms of transport—it may be too late. Aim to descend to below the altitude at which the patient last felt well when waking in the morning. A descent of as little as 450–900m may be sufficient. Do not continue to ascend if symptomatic, and when recovered and ready to re-ascend, do so cautiously.

Antiemetics/pain relief Use domperidone, cyclizine or ondansetron to treat sickness. Avoid antiemetics that are sedating, such as promethazine. Use acetaminophen, ibuprofen or diclofenac for pain relief, and avoid sedating painkillers, such as morphine.

Dexamethasone Use for severe AMS and HACE. Give dexamethasone 8mg orally, IV, or IM immediately, followed by 4mg every 6 hours.

Acetazolamide Use for the treatment of AMS, HACE and HAPE. Give acetazolamide 250mg orally three times daily. It may not be possible to give this drug to patients who are breathless or to those who have reduced consciousness. Acetazolamide can also be used to prevent AMS (*see* below).

Nifedipine Use for the treatment of HAPE. Give nifedipine 10mg immediately, followed by 20–30mg (of the slow release form) every 12 hours until there are no symptoms and you are at lower altitude. Monitor blood pressure, as nifedipine may significantly lower the blood pressure, particularly in the presence of trauma or hypothermia.

Albuterol (an inhaled Beta-2 agonist) Use to treat HAPE: 2 puffs every 6 hours. May be delivered using a spacer for patients who are very short of breath.

Hyperbaric therapy Use for the treatment of AMS, HACE and HAPE. Use for 2–6 hours or more until symptoms relieved, then descend. May require repeated treatments until descent arranged. Can be used with supplemental oxygen. Take care of airway if conscious level is reduced. *See* p.61 for types of portable hyperbaric bags.

Other altitude disorders

Sleep disturbance
Disturbed sleep is common on ascent to altitude and may cause fatigue.

Symptoms and Signs	Treatment
□ Frequent awakening □ Periodic breathing □ Potentially worse at higher altitude	□ May require longer periods of rest □ Use of "sleeping pills" such as temazepam under medical direction only □ Acetazolamide 125mg in the evening may help

Periodic breathing
This term refers to periods of faster breathing with intervals of no breathing. The individual may wake with the feeling of suffocation, which can be unsettling.

Symptoms and Signs	Treatment
□ Episodes of faster breathing followed by no breathing □ May be followed by gasps or rapid deep breaths □ Cycle repeated over 5–10 minutes □ May be associated with oxygen saturations below 60%	□ May require longer periods of rest □ Use of "sleeping pills" such as temazepam under medical direction only □ Acetazolamide 125mg in the evening may help. Increase the dose to 250mg if necessary.

Persistent cough (bronchitis/pharyngitis)

A tickling persistent cough with dry throat is very common at altitude and can be extremely irritating. Occasionally it may be a sign of an underlying chest infection that requires treatment with antibiotics.

Symptoms and signs	Treatment
□ Dry, sore throat □ Dry, sore nasal passages □ Persistent cough, usually dry □ Sputum that may become yellow/green □ Temperature	□ Throat antiseptic and local anesthetic lozenges □ Maintain good hydration □ Albuterol inhaler 2 puffs four times a day may help cough □ Nasal ointments (mupirocin, petroleum jelly) □ If yellow sputum, high temperature, unwell, will need antibiotics

Peripheral edema

More irritating and uncomfortable than harmful. Swelling of ankles and feet may cause occasional problems with footwear and blisters. Occasionally a sign of the onset of AMS, HACE and HAPE; watch for deterioration and monitor closely.

Symptoms and signs	Treatment
□ Swelling of fingers, hands, toes, feet and face, especially around the eyes □ Rings and shoes may be tight □ Facial swelling is obvious to others □ More common in females □ May precede AMS etc.	□ No treatment unless impeding physical performance □ May require descent by 450-900m or several rest days □ Acetazolamide 125mg or 250mg orally twice daily

Snow blindness

This condition is similar to sea blindness or corneal flash burns. It is caused by sunburn of the eye by UV rays and is a particular risk on snow due to surface reflection.

Symptoms and signs	Treatment
□ May happen after only 2-3 hours exposure □ Very painful, gritty, red eyes □ Face may be burnt red as well □ Bright light may hurt eye □ Headache is common □ Usually both eyes affected □ Eyelids may be swollen	□ Prevention is best—sunglasses with good protection from the sides □ Assess for foreign bodies □ Local anesthetic drops for pain, and oral painkillers for headache □ Antibiotic ointment may lubricate the eyes and help to relieve pain □ Use eye patch for 24 hours then reassess (not if discharging)

5 Portable hyperbaric chamber

This is a flexible bag made of durable material, with a manual pump and a blow-off valve. The casualty is put inside and the bag pressurized using the pump. This quickly provides an effective drop in altitude of approximately 2,000m. Supplementary oxygen can be used. The disadvantages are that monitoring an unconscious casualty is difficult and that continual pumping is exhausting but absolutely necessary to maintain pressure and clear carbon dioxide breathed out by the casualty.
Three brands are available:
□ Gamow™ Bags
□ Certec Caisson™
□ PAC™ (Portable Altitude Chamber)

6 Pulse oximeters

These devices are compact and fit on the end of a finger. By shining a light through the finger end, they detect the amount of oxygen in the blood and the pulse rate. They are very useful and provide objective information that is essential in treating a casualty at altitude.
There are many makes; here is a selection:
□ Merlin™ Medical Impulse Finger Oximeter
□ Nonin™ Onyx Finger Oximeter
□ Smiths Medical™ OXI-PULSE 3520 Finger Oximeter

Prevention of high altitude illnesses

□ Spend at least one to two nights at 2,400m on the way up.
□ Ascend only approximately 400–600m per day.
□ Climb high during the day and descend to sleep.
□ Maintain good hydration, rest and nutrition.
□ Avoid extreme exercise.
□ Avoid alcohol and sedative drugs.
□ Use acetazolamide:
  – Take 250mg twice daily
  – Start at least 24 hours before ascent
  – Watch for allergic reactions
  – Side effects include tingling fingers, altered taste, passing large amounts of urine, nausea and diarrhea.

Risk factors for high altitude illnesses

□ Previous episode(s) of high altitude illness
□ Rate of ascent
□ Absolute altitude
□ Extreme exercise
□ Pre-existing chest infections
□ Chronic cardiac or pulmonary disease

Anticipate, Prevent, Recognize, Descend

COLD CLIMATES

The ability of humans to adapt and survive unsupported in a cold environment is very limited, so expeditions to areas of extreme cold present a special challenge. Survival depends upon correct behavior and equipment and prompt action if things go wrong.

The onset of cold injuries and hypothermia can cause slow deterioration of physical and mental function that goes unnoticed by the casualty. Mutual dependence among members of the expedition will reduce the risk of serious injury and illness. The best way to stay warm is to limit the loss of body heat.

Wind chill factor and time to frostbite

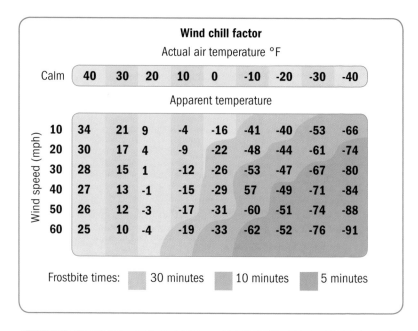

Wind chill factor

Actual air temperature °F

Calm	40	30	20	10	0	-10	-20	-30	-40

Apparent temperature

Wind speed (mph)	40	30	20	10	0	-10	-20	-30	-40
10	34	21	9	-4	-16	-41	-40	-53	-66
20	30	17	4	-9	-22	-48	-44	-61	-74
30	28	15	1	-12	-26	-53	-47	-67	-80
40	27	13	-1	-15	-29	57	-49	-71	-84
50	26	12	-3	-17	-31	-60	-51	-74	-88
60	25	10	-4	-19	-33	-62	-52	-76	-91

Frostbite times: ▢ 30 minutes ▢ 10 minutes ▢ 5 minutes

Factors exacerbating cold injury and hypothermia

- Cold temperature
- Damp/wet
- Windchill
- Sweating during work
- Drugs/alcohol
- Sickness
- Dehydration
- Lack of food
- Lack of sleep
- Injury

Prevention strategy

- Clothing
  - Dry, warm, suitable for conditions
  - Hat, gloves, mitts, face protection
  - Dry boots, not tight
- Good nutrition
- Hydration
- Limit outdoor exposure time
- Use heater if possible
- Avoid alcohol
- Get good rest

Cold injury

Nonfreezing injury precedes freezing injury and may occur at temperatures above 32°F (0°C) (ignoring wind chill), so be vigilant. Freezing injury happens faster below -15°F (-26°C) and may occur after less than two minutes of exposure.

Chilblains and "sausage" fingers

Symptoms and signs	Treatment
□ Small, itchy, red, shiny lumps on fingers and toes □ Thickened skin, reduced sensation	□ Keep extremities warm, dry □ Painkillers if sore □ Avoid delicate jobs

Polar hands

Symptoms and signs	Treatment
□ Painful fissures in the skin around the fingertips and nails □ May affect balls and heels of feet □ If red and sore, likely to be infected	□ Regular moisturizer □ Keep clean with antiseptic solution □ Antibiotic ointment for infection □ Tape or glue fissures together

Trench feet

Symptoms and signs	Treatment
□ Cold, wet feet in tight boots □ Cold, pale skin, reduced sensation □ Painful on rewarming	□ Dry, loose-fitting boots and socks □ Warm and dry feet when possible □ Do not let boots freeze when off

Frostnip

Symptoms and signs	Treatment
□ Initially painless □ Small (5mm) white, cold, firm areas □ Affects fingers, ears, nose tip, feet □ Exacerbated by contact with metal—facial piercings, glasses	□ Be vigilant about the risk □ Simple warming techniques □ May be painful on rewarming □ Do not rub—increases tissue damage and swelling

Frostbite

Symptoms and signs	Treatment
□ Develops from frostnip in minutes □ Waxy white or even black □ Numb and stiff □ Possible swelling of extremity or limb □ May blister on rewarming—leave blisters intact	□ Bathe in water at 104°F (40°C) □ Give oxygen if at altitude □ Dress with sterile dressing □ Keep elevated, warm, dry □ Painkillers, antibiotics □ Get medical advice urgently

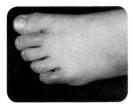

Chilblains

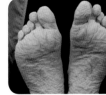

Trench feet

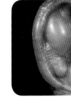

Frostbite

Hypothermia

The onset of hypothermia may be insidious and go unnoticed until the body core temperature has dropped significantly—the casualty may be lethargic, confused and withdrawn. This state is extremely dangerous and may lead to accidents.

Mild hypothermia
Core (rectal) temperature: 98.6°F (37°C)—normal—to 95°F (35°C)

Symptoms and signs	Treatment
□ Shivering, cold to touch □ Numb hands and feet □ Becoming lethargic and slightly confused □ Decision making may be impaired □ May be irritable, denying there is any problem	□ Shelter in tent, snow hole, wind break. Huddle with team members □ Use dry clothes,dry sleeping bags, survival bag, hat, mittens □ Insulate from ground with sleeping mats, rucksacks, vegetation □ Give warm, sweet drinks, food □ Rest until warm and not shivering

Moderate hypothermia
Core (rectal) temperature: 95°F (35°C) to 90°F (32.2°C)

Symptoms and signs	Treatment
□ A reduction in conscious level, confused, disorientated □ Uncoordinated, stumbling, falling □ Very sleepy, lethargic □ Shivering has stopped □ Stiff muscles □ Increasing risk of arrhythmias (abnormal heart beat) □ Inability to raise core temperature	□ Urgent action: call for medical advice □ Alert whole group and focus □ Make a shelter for everyone (if one has hypothermia, others may follow) □ Handle casualty carefully to avoid triggering arrhythmias □ Pair together in sleeping bags □ Keep in recovery position □ Monitor pulse and breathing

Severe hypothermia
Core (rectal) temperature: below 88°F (31.1°C)

Symptoms and signs	Treatment
□ Unconscious □ Very pale or blue □ Breathing and pulse may be very slow or hard to detect (see p.180-181 on taking pulse) □ Rigid muscles □ Pupils may be dilated and unresponsive	□ Seek medical advice and evacuate □ Handle casualty as for a spinal patient (see p.96-97) □ Breathing/pulse: recovery position, rewarm, and monitor (see p.27) □ No pulse: start CPR, try to reach core temperature >90°F (32.2°C). Seek medical advice, see p.28

Chronic conditions worsened by cold climates

Asthma Cold air is a potent trigger of asthma attacks, even in those not known to suffer from asthma. Heavy exercise is another trigger, and the two together may induce a severe attack. Known sufferers should be aware of the risks and a treatment plan should be in place.

Angina Known sufferers of angina may find that in the cold, chest pain is provoked by less physical exercise than normal. They may even get chest pain at rest, which is a medical emergency (*see* p.46). Chest pain in others may be caused by previously covert heart disease and should be treated accordingly (*see* p.146). Known sufferers should be wary of venturing in to the extreme cold.

Raynaud's disease Cold is a potent trigger of severe peripheral vasoconstriction, which reduces finger functionality. Fingers are then very painful on rewarming. Hand warmers, medications such as nifedipine, painkillers and avoidance of cold will limit severity of attacks. Raynauds is associated with other serious diseases. A detailed medical history should be obtained before departure.

Some other diseases (such as peripheral vascular disease and cold agglutinin disease) may be dangerously exacerbated by extreme cold. Seek medical advice before departure.

Children and cold climates

Surface to volume ratio This is greater in children—they lose body heat faster

Activity Children may be carried in back packs, on sledges or on skidoos at speed. Being inactive, they generate less body heat and may rapidly become hypothermic. Lower limbs are particularly at risk in a back pack due to constriction around the upper thigh, increasing the risk of cold injury.

Communication Children may not describe cold but become grumpy or quiet. Be alert to possible drop in temperature. Check warmth and circulation (*see* p.181).

Food and drink Proportionally more is required by children and at frequent, regular intervals. This will maintain equanimity!

Clothing for cold climates

Attire must be robust and fit for purpose. Wear three layers and shed outer layers when working to avoid overheating. Replace outer layers when not active.

Inner layer Thin "thermals" with long arms and legs. Natural material such as merino wool or silk have good moisture wicking properties and can be worn for many days without washing. Synthetic fibers based on olefin (polypropylene, polyolefin), such as Hollofil™ and Capilene™, are also effective.

Mid-layer Thicker layer, adding insulation, high neck for top. Fleece (made from polyester fibers) and Thinsulate™ are effective. Wool has good insulating properties, but is difficult to dry if wet (for example, from sweat). Down is warm and packs small, but loses insulation significantly when wet.

Outer layer This may be two parts incorporating a down (or synthetic lofting) jacket with outer shell and pants. The outer shell should be breathable (eg Gore-Tex™) with the possibility of opening vents for increased ventilation, have an adjustable hood, pockets accessible with backpack in place, bright color and high neck closure. Pants should also be breathable, with long zips up the sides to enable donning without removal of boots.

Hands, feet Mitts are warmer than gloves, and a "shell" system can be used. Take spares. Socks may be wool or synthetic "ragg" style. Gaiters prevent ingress of snow and should be reinforced on the medial side to prevent chafe. Overboots may be required in the extreme cold.

Head and face An uncovered head can result in 70% heat loss. Use a balaclava and face mask if conditions worsen. The hat must be able to cover the ears if necessary. May be made from wool or synthetic fiber. Take extras.

HOT CLIMATES

Hot climates, whether scorching dry deserts or humid tropical rain forests, present humans with severe challenges. The body has a greater ability to acclimatize to hot climates than to extreme cold, but the process may take 10 to 20 days.

A combination of high humidity (which prevents the heat loss brought on by sweating), lack of acclimatization, high work rate, and predisposing factors may precipitate heat illness—not necessarily extreme temperature.

Desert climates present the twofold problem of extreme heat during the day and severe cold (even below-zero temperatures) at night. Tropical rain forests, on the other hand, have very high rainfall and humidity, which causes problems with the increased incidence of infections. They also harbor a high prevalence of unwelcome insects and other animals (see p.80–83).

Hyperthermia

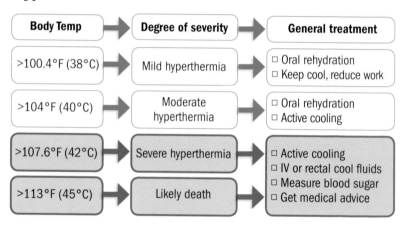

Body Temp	Degree of severity	General treatment
>100.4°F (38°C)	Mild hyperthermia	□ Oral rehydration □ Keep cool, reduce work
>104°F (40°C)	Moderate hyperthermia	□ Oral rehydration □ Active cooling
>107.6°F (42°C)	Severe hyperthermia	□ Active cooling □ IV or rectal cool fluids □ Measure blood sugar □ Get medical advice
>113°F (45°C)	Likely death	

Risk factors for hyperthermia and heat illness

Human factors
- □ Dehydration (diarrhea, menstruation)
- □ Diabetes
- □ Lack of sleep
- □ Reduced food intake
- □ Fever, infection
- □ Old age
- □ Sunburn
- □ Alcohol

Environmental factors
- □ Increased air temperature
- □ Increased humidity
- □ Increased solar heat
- □ Decreased wind speed

Work load
- □ Working at near-maximum heart rate for long periods

Medication
- □ Beta blockers
- □ Diuretics
- □ Amphetamines
- □ Cocaine/ecstasy
- □ Prochlorperazine
- □ Tricyclic antidepressants
- □ Theophylline
- □ Anticholinergics (atropine, scopolamine)
- □ Antihistamines

Prevention of heat illnesses

- □ Plan expedition to allow time for acclimatization
- □ Identify those at risk (see previous page)
- □ Take care with previous sufferers
- □ Team approach to rehydration
- □ Monitor work rate
- □ Recognize symptoms early
- □ Monitor weather conditions (heat and humidity) and plan activities accordingly
- □ Have adequate clothing and shade

Specific heat illnesses

> It is crucial to remember, and consider, that a high temperature and/or collapse may not necessarily be due to a heat-related illness.

Sunburn—see p.166

Heat cramps
Possibly due to lack of salts in diet or increase in salt losses by sweat

Symptoms and signs	Treatment
□ Usually leg cramps during or after exercise □ Patient may be fit and acclimatized	□ Salt replacement drink to rehydrate □ Increase regular salt intake with food while in hot climate

Prickly heat (miliaria rubra)
Blocked, inflamed, infected sweat glands which then cannot function to cool the body.

Symptoms and signs

- □ Red, raised, itchy spots or blisters on skin usually covered by clothing (hands usually spared)
- □ May become infected: boils, spots
- □ Blocked sweat glands

Treatment

- □ Keep skin clean with good hygiene
- □ Keep cool, reduce work load
- □ Relieve itching (chlorpheniramine)
- □ Antibiotics may be needed for infected skin (mupirocin or dicloxacillin)

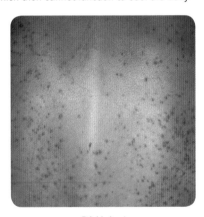

Prickly heat

Heat syncope
Dilated blood vessels in the lower body leads to a decrease in blood pressure, causing a reduction in blood flow to the brain, leading to collapse.

Symptoms and signs	Treatment
□ Sudden fainting on rising from sitting position □ May be lightheaded before collapse □ Usually quick recovery	□ Recovery position in the shade □ Salt replacement drink (see p.185) □ **Consider heat exhaustion or stroke if no quick recovery**

Heat exhaustion

Exhaustion secondary to water and salt loss caused by sweating. Several liters may be lost. Temperature may only be slightly raised.

Symptoms and signs	Treatment
□ Heavy sweating □ Very little, dark urine output □ Lethargic weak, low blood pressure □ Muscle cramps □ Temperature normal or slightly raised □ Rapid pulse/breathing □ Loss of consciousness	□ Move to cool shade, lay down □ Cool with wet covers and fanning □ Salt replacement drink (see p.185) □ IV or rectal route (see p.184) if unconscious □ Consider heat stroke if unconscious; seek medical advice

Heat stroke

This is an emergency, and may cause death. Seek medical advice immediately. Core temp >104°F (40°C). Reduced sweating, prickly heat, not acclimatized.

Symptoms and signs	Treatment
□ Hot, dry skin (may not be sweating) □ Headache □ Nausea, vomiting □ Weakness, staggering □ Anxiety, confusion, restlessness □ Low blood sugar, seizures □ Loss of consciousness	□ Move to shade, lay down □ Cool with wet covers, ice packs in groin and armpits, fanning □ Cool IV or rectal fluids (see p.184): 1L initially □ Measure blood sugar—correct if low □ Seek medical advice

Hyponatremia (low sodium level in the blood)

Hyponatremia usually follows heavy sweating with excess sodium loss followed by rehydration with plain water. However, a large intake of plain water (more than 4L) may cause symptomatic hyponatremia without sweating. Medications such as diuretics may cause severe hyponatremia.

Symptoms and signs	Treatment
□ May have good urine output □ Weakness, lethargy, muscle cramps □ Dizziness, unsteady on feet □ Nausea, vomiting □ Confusion, agitation □ Seizures, loss of consciousness	□ **Unconscious: seek medical advice immediately** (see p.34-36) □ Treat seizures—see p.38 □ Do not give further water □ Conscious: give salty food □ Casualty may require IV fluids (0.9% saline solution) to correct the low sodium level. This treatment is highly specialized: have medical advice on hand before and during administration

See p.184 for rehydration techniques

Wounds and fungal infections

In hot and humid climates, there is greater risk of a wound becoming infected with either skin organisms or new organisms from the surrounding environment. Take the risk of infection seriously; an infected wound takes much longer to heal.

- ☐ Clean the wound with 2% chlorhexidine, iodine solution or dry iodine spray.
- ☐ Cover the wound with an occlusive sterile dressing.
- ☐ Try to keep as dry as possible and inspect and clean daily.
- ☐ If pus in the wound or spreading redness in the skin around the wound (cellulitis), give antibiotics (such as amoxicillin + clavulanate, dicloxacillin or erythromycin).

Fungal infections of the groin, underneath the breast, in the armpits and between the toes are a common problem in hot and humid climates. Be vigilant about a spreading reddish rash in these areas. The skin may crack between the toes and be very painful. See p.166 for the treatment of skin infections.

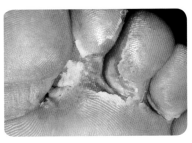

Athlete's foot

- ☐ Keep these areas as dry as possible and clean thoroughly and frequently.
- ☐ Use dry socks/footwear when possible.
- ☐ Treat suspected infections with an antifungal agent (such as miconazole 2% cream or powder).

Acclimatization

Most humans (but not all) can acclimatize to a hot environment in 10–20 days. A greater amount of exercise (up to 2 hours per day of strenuous exercise, raising the heart rate to 2/3 of theoretical maximum) speeds up acclimatization, but avoid excercise in the hottest part of the day. People with a larger body mass index and those who are less fit will have less capacity to acclimatize.

Advantages	Disadvantages
☐ Increased capacity for exercise ☐ Increased sweat production which lowers body temperature at a given exercise rate ☐ Sweating starts at a lower core body temperature ☐ Decreased sodium loss in sweat ☐ Decreased sodium loss in urine	☐ Increased fluid loss per hour requiring increased balanced fluid intake to avoid dehydration ☐ Acclimatization may be less effective in humid environments, so reduce exercise rate to avoid overheating ☐ Thirst is a late sign of dehydration. Take on fluid before thirst starts.

Taking the temperature

Oral temperature readings are usually more accurate than those taken in the armpit. Be very careful if the casualty is unconscious. The thermometer must be firmly under the tongue for two minutes, with no mouth breathing. Ear thermometers are more prone to user error but are reasonably accurate if used correctly.

Rectal temperatures may be inaccurate if there are feces in the rectum and take some time to equalize with the body core temperature.

MARINE AND INLAND WATERS

Inland waters such as rivers and lakes may be considerable bodies of water and tend to be cold. Marine waters tend to be warmer but most are under 75–80°F (24–27°C), which can cause hypothermia.

Immersion and drowning

Immersion causes several responses in the body. In addition, a sudden illness (such as a heart attack) may have caused the fall into the water, or the fall may have caused injury. Falls in to fast flowing rivers carry the very real risk of significant injury.

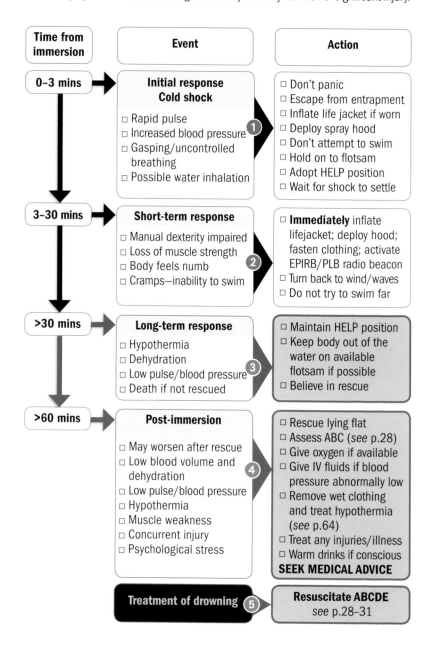

Time from immersion	Event	Action
0–3 mins	**Initial response Cold shock** ① □ Rapid pulse □ Increased blood pressure □ Gasping/uncontrolled breathing □ Possible water inhalation	□ Don't panic □ Escape from entrapment □ Inflate life jacket if worn □ Deploy spray hood □ Don't attempt to swim □ Hold on to flotsam □ Adopt HELP position □ Wait for shock to settle
3–30 mins	**Short-term response** ② □ Manual dexterity impaired □ Loss of muscle strength □ Body feels numb □ Cramps—inability to swim	□ **Immediately** inflate lifejacket; deploy hood; fasten clothing; activate EPIRB/PLB radio beacon □ Turn back to wind/waves □ Do not try to swim far
>30 mins	**Long-term response** ③ □ Hypothermia □ Dehydration □ Low pulse/blood pressure □ Death if not rescued	□ Maintain HELP position □ Keep body out of the water on available flotsam if possible □ Believe in rescue
>60 mins	**Post-immersion** ④ □ May worsen after rescue □ Low blood volume and dehydration □ Low pulse/blood pressure □ Hypothermia □ Muscle weakness □ Concurrent injury □ Psychological stress	□ Rescue lying flat □ Assess ABC (see p.28) □ Give oxygen if available □ Give IV fluids if blood pressure abnormally low □ Remove wet clothing and treat hypothermia (see p.64) □ Treat any injuries/illness □ Warm drinks if conscious **SEEK MEDICAL ADVICE**
	Treatment of drowning ⑤	**Resuscitate ABCDE** see p.28–31

1 Initial response: Cold shock (0–3 minutes)

Respiration becomes rapid and gasping, and the abrupt increase in blood pressure may precipitate a heart attack or stroke in the vulnerable. Wait for the effects of sudden immersion to settle, which should happen in a few minutes. Holding onto available flotsam will have a stabilizing and reassuring effect.

2 Short term response (3–30 minutes)

Manual dexterity will quickly become impaired, so complete all essential tasks immediately. Water exerts a "squeeze" on the body, causing dehydration and the possibility of circulatory collapse on being rescued. Get as much of the body onto flotsam as possible, to minimize heat loss. Maintain HELP position (Heat Escape Lessening Position), and bunch up close with any others

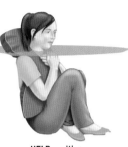

HELP position

3 Long term response (30 minutes and longer)

The onset of hypothermia is swift, especially in colder water, and may be fatal if rescue is delayed (for treatment see p.64). Believe you will be rescued, but leave the rescuing to the rescuers, and do not attempt to swim any distance yourself.

4 Post-immersion response (60 minutes and longer)

It is well known that a casualty may collapse at the time of rescue or shortly afterwards (circum-rescue collapse). This is due to several factors:

□ Loss of hydrostatic support to the lower body, causing circulatory collapse on removal from the water, exacerbated by dehydration
□ Acute lung injury caused by a significant amount of water (salt or fresh) in the lungs
□ Profound hypothermia
□ Underlying injury or illness.

The main elements of treatment are to resuscitate the casualty if unconscious (see p.28-29), treat the hypothermia (see p.64) and monitor pulse, blood pressure, respiration and level of consciousness. Watch for signs of deterioration. It is vital to check for injuries. Most importantly, **seek medical advice at an early stage**.

5 Treatment of drowning

□ Assess ABCDE immediately (see p.28-31)–**start with 5 rescue breaths**.
□ Do not waste time trying to empty water from the lungs.
□ The casualty may have water in the stomach and may vomit. If vomiting occurs, turn the casualty onto one side and clear the mouth of vomit to protect the airway.
□ Treat hypothermia (see p.64) and keep casualty as dry and warm as possible.
□ Continue resuscitating until the casualty has a temperature greater than 90°F (32.2°C) and is breathing, medical help arrives, or you are exhausted and must stop.

Acute lung injury may affect breathing over the next 24-48 hours, causing shortness of breath/fast breathing, coughing, rapid pulse and possible collapse. If water has entered the lungs, give oxygen if available and evacuate. **Seek medical advice early.**

FOOD AND WATER

An army marches on its stomach, and an expedition is little different. To maintain a high physical work rate, it is essential to keep fuel and hydration levels high. This applies particularly to children, who will suddenly run out of energy and then stop if they are not kept fed and hydrated (see p.18–19).

On a short expedition, it is possible to take all the food and water you will need with you, but longer trips will require some local provision, and care must be taken to avoid infections of the stomach and gut.

Water and energy requirements:

70kg person in a temperate climate

At rest	1500–2000 kcal/day
	2.5–3.5L water/day
Moderate work	2000–5000 kcal/day
(hiking over rough ground for several hours/day)	4–6L water/day
Heavy work	5000–7500 kcal/day
(hiking carrying significant loads for several hours a day)	6–15L water/day
Very heavy work in cold environments	>8000 kcal/day
(hauling sledge for many hours a day)	10–15L+ water/day

Some important points regarding these figures:
☐ They are only very broad guidelines, and each person should assess their individual calorie and fluid intake.
☐ Hot climates will increase fluid requirements markedly.
☐ Cold climates will increase calorie requirements markedly.
☐ Rehydration should not only be with plain water but should also contain salt replacement.
☐ These figures can be used to calculate overall food and water requirements for an expedition, but a contingency should also be included.
☐ The figures for water requirements apply to solely personal direct consumption. Allow 2–4L per day per person for cooking, cleaning teeth etc.

Survival requirements

During survival conditions in the wilderness, the most important requirement is water. The body will require an absolute minimum of 1.5L to maintain equilibrium in a temperate climate while sedentary. Never drink seawater or urine (your own or anyone else's), as this will increase body dehydration. See p.86 for water collection techniques.

A person can survive for many days without food, but physical reserve will decrease as fat reserves are used, and muscle is then resorbed by the body.

Food poisoning and gut infections

Disabling diarrhea and vomiting are common on expeditions. These symptoms are usually due to food poisoning, but it is important to consider alternative diagnoses (see p.151). The time course will give an idea as to diagnosis and hence treatment.

Diagnosis	Time to peak illness (days)	Severity of vomiting or diarrhea	Fever	Time to resolution (days)
Food poisoning	1-2	Very severe	No	2-3
Bacterial infection	2-4	Severe	Yes	5-12
Protozoa (Giardia)	Variable course	Severe	Yes	5-12

Treatment of food poisoning and gut infections
☐ Rehydrate, aiming for several urinations per day of pale urine.
☐ If severe, consider ciprofloxacin 1000mg on day one. Following the first dose, continue ciprofloxacin 500mg twice daily for three days if symptoms persist.
☐ If symptoms persist despite ciprofloxacin, treat with metronidazole or tinidazole (cause may be other infective organisms such as protozoa or other bacteria).
☐ If required by circumstances (currently climbing, at very high altitude, in camp but storm-bound) consider loperamide to limit diarrhea (see p.151).
☐ Evacuate if IV fluids are required, diarrhea is bloody, casualty has high fever (>104°F, or 40°C) or symptoms persist for longer than 4 days.

Food

Rules for using locally-sourced food
☐ "If you can't wash it, peel it, or boil it, forget it"—global proverb.
☐ Clean and peel all fruit and vegetables thoroughly in purified drinking water— this may still not remove all risk of poisoning.
☐ Avoid salads and dairy-based items, such as untreated milk, if possible.

Rules for food preparation
☐ Anyone unwell with diarrhea, vomiting or fever should not handle food.
☐ Clean hands thoroughly before and after preparing food. Alcohol hand gels and antibacterial handwash products are useful.
☐ Clean preparation area thoroughly. Antibacterial surface cleaner is valuable.
☐ Use separate boards and utensils for meat and vegetables.
☐ Cook thoroughly and avoid contamination after cooking (wash plates, utensils etc).
☐ Food should not be recooked/reheated.
☐ Dispose of all food waste immediately and away from preparation area.

Storage
☐ Use air- and moisture-tight, clearly labeled containers.
☐ Use waterproof labels that won't come off and permanent marker pen.
☐ Store away from insect infestation, rodents and other large animals such as bears.
☐ Store in logical sequence so the food to be used first is accessible. Box food in units of "day" and "week" consumption.

Types of food suitable for expeditions

Food type	Advantages	Disadvantages
Freeze dried	□ Convenient to use □ Light to transport □ Easy to prepare □ Easy to pack	□ Risk of severe constipation if not properly rehydrated □ Can be monotonous every day. Needs drinking quality water for preparation
Boil-in-bag	□ Convenient to use □ Can eat direct from the bag □ High fluid content □ Easy to prepare—can boil in untreated water but take care with contamination	□ Heavy to transport □ Can be monotonous every day
Tinned	□ Convenient to use □ Can eat direct from the tin □ High fluid content □ Secure from infection	□ Heavy to transport □ Disposal of empty tins □ Paper labels may come off
Dry produce	□ Light to transport □ Good variety—encourages high food intake	□ Risk of contamination, infestation □ Easily ruined by water ingress □ More difficult to prepare

Food allergies and intolerance

Most expedition members will already know about any food allergies and intolerances they may have. However, new reactions may come to light, and local processed food may not be labeled accurately.

Although an individual can be allergic to any type of food, the following foods account for 90 percent of food allergies:

□ Nuts □ Fish □ Shellfish
□ Dairy products □ Eggs □ Soy

Many of these products are incorporated in to the processing of other food types—for example, soybeans and soy products are found in baked goods, canned tuna, cereals, crackers, infant formulas, sauces and soups—so care should be taken to check contents as thoroughly as possible.

Food intolerance, unlike food allergy, does not involve the immune system and is not life-threatening. Lactose intolerance—trouble digesting the milk sugar lactose—is one example. Symptoms may include stomach cramps, bloating and diarrhea.

Known sufferers of severe allergies should take ample supplies of anti-allergy medications with them to wilderness areas and the team's medical kit should contain a general stock for unsuspected reactions. See p.48–49 for the emergency treatment of allergic reactions.

Water

It is usually not possible to transport all the water that will be required for an expedition. Therefore water must be sourced locally, and this must be done carefully. It is prudent to treat all water from whatever source, even the most pristine mountain stream.

Sources of local water

Streams and springs	Make sure stream is away from human habitation—the higher the better. Check for dead animals etc.
Rainwater	Use a cleaned and treated surface for collection and keep tanks sealed. It is wise to treat also.
Wells	May be contaminated through the groundwater table and percolating sewage. Treat as heavily contaminated.
Rivers	Less wise, as one of the many sources of water feeding the river may be contaminated.
Lakes	Still or stagnant water, especially round the edges, may be contaminated. Avoid if possible.
Snow/ice	A considerable amount of fuel is required to melt snow and ice. Ice is more effective. The salt content of the upper layers of sea ice is lowest. Taste it to check for salinity.

Water treatment (purification and disinfection)

☐ Purification—the removal of inorganic material, such as silt, and organic material, such as framents of vegetation.
☐ Disinfection—the removal or destruction of harmful micro-organisms such as bacteria, protozoa and viruses.

Purification

Filtration	Effective. Various types of filter available (Millbank bag, mechanical filters). Charcoal stages may be incorporated in some filters, which improves taste. Flow rate is relatively low, so the filter needs to run continually to provide sufficient water. Some micro-organisms will pass through.
Settling	Takes time, and large storage capacity is required. Very fine suspended particles take days to settle completely.
Coagulation/flocculation	Removes suspended particles including most micro-organisms by aggregation. Resultant larger particles settle faster and are more easily filtered. Alum is the chemical most commonly used for this process.

Disinfection

Note that treatment with iodine or chlorine does not remove cryptosporidium, which should be removed by filtration, boiling or another method.

Boiling	Rolling boil for 1 minute at sea level. At 6,000m, water boils at about 175°F (80°C), so boil for 3 minutes. Cover while cooling.
Iodine disinfection: (1 drop or 0.05ml)	Several forms of iodine may be used: – 2% iodine solution: 5 drops/l (double if giardia suspected) – Lugols' solution: 4 drops/l – Saturated solution of iodine crystals in water: 10–15ml/l – Iodine tablets are also available. Crush before using. □ Leave any water for a minimum of 30 minutes before using. □ Ascorbic acid (vitamin C) will improve taste after iodine use. □ Iodine treated water is not recommended for pregnant women, people with thyroid disease, or use for over 2-3 months.
Chlorine disinfection	□ Commercial products (tablets, solution, powder) are available. □ The effectiveness of chlorine is reduced by cold, organic matter, and alkaline water—should be left for longer after treatment. □ Taste is better with iodine, but sodium thiosulfate can also be used with chlorine to improve taste. □ Can be used in people with thyroid problems.
Mechanical filters	□ A viable field alternative, but can be heavy and expensive. □ Small one-use filters can be incorporated into drinking bottles, but sometimes the water requires further treatment. □ Some incorporate charcoal filters and iodine resin.
Reverse osmosis filters	□ Commonly used on boats, for desalination of seawater (run from boat power source or hand-powered). □ Removes all contaminants from treated water. □ Very effective but difficult to transport and labor intensive.

Water storage

The key is to prevent recontamination once water has been purified and disinfected. Seal storage containers and tanks to prevent gross contamination. Plastic tanks in 10–20L volumes, fitted with taps, are convenient and portable.

If chlorine has been used for initial disinfection, the residual chlorine will provide some protection against recontamination for a day or so. For longer term storage, pretreatment with chlorine (calcium hypochlorite mixed in solution with hydrogen peroxide) will maintain water in good condition. Dechlorinate immediately prior to use.

Water on the move

□ By vehicle: avoid storing all of your water in one container or tank. If it ruptures, there is no "Plan B." Plastic tanks may wear through but are light, while metal tanks are more robust, but heavy. Do not stow water on the roof, but place it low in the vehicle, thereby increasing stability by lowering the center of gravity.

□ On foot: for personal use to maintain hydration, water bladders (such as the Camelbak™) are very useful. Up to 5L can be incorporated into backpacks and enable continual hydration while exercising. Ensure they are cleaned after every use, particularly if sugar-containing solutions have been used, avoiding contamination with untreated water.

PLANTS AND FUNGI

Some plants and fungi are poisonous and can cause unpleasant, even life-threatening problems (such as anaphylaxis) after contact or ingestion. Identification is not always possible, so treat symptoms.

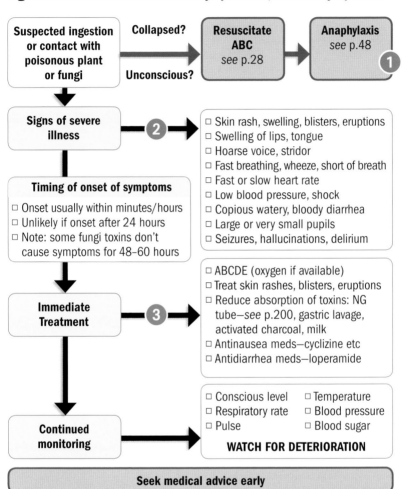

Suspected ingestion or contact with poisonous plant or fungi	Collapsed? Unconscious?	**Resuscitate ABC** *see p.28* → **Anaphylaxis** *see p.48* ①

Signs of severe illness ②
→ ☐ Skin rash, swelling, blisters, eruptions
☐ Swelling of lips, tongue
☐ Hoarse voice, stridor
☐ Fast breathing, wheeze, short of breath
☐ Fast or slow heart rate
☐ Low blood pressure, shock
☐ Copious watery, bloody diarrhea
☐ Large or very small pupils
☐ Seizures, hallucinations, delirium

Timing of onset of symptoms
☐ Onset usually within minutes/hours
☐ Unlikely if onset after 24 hours
☐ Note: some fungi toxins don't cause symptoms for 48-60 hours

Immediate Treatment ③
→ ☐ ABCDE (oxygen if available)
☐ Treat skin rashes, blisters, eruptions
☐ Reduce absorption of toxins: NG tube—*see p.200*, gastric lavage, activated charcoal, milk
☐ Antinausea meds—cyclizine etc
☐ Antidiarrhea meds—loperamide

Continued monitoring
→ ☐ Conscious level ☐ Temperature
☐ Respiratory rate ☐ Blood pressure
☐ Pulse ☐ Blood sugar
WATCH FOR DETERIORATION

Seek medical advice early

① Anaphylaxis

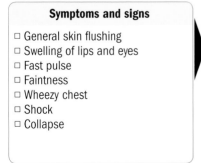

Symptoms and signs	Treatment
☐ General skin flushing ☐ Swelling of lips and eyes ☐ Fast pulse ☐ Faintness ☐ Wheezy chest ☐ Shock ☐ Collapse	☐ ABCDE if collapsed ☐ Epinephrine 0.5mg IM (0.5ml of 1:1000 solution) ☐ Antihistamine: chlorpheniramine 10-20mg IM ☐ Steroid: hydrocortisone 100mg IM/IV ☐ IV fluids (500ml immediately) ☐ Further treatment—*see p.48-49*

2 Signs of severe illness

Observation	Danger signs
Conscious state and orientation	□ Reduced conscious state (see p.37-38) □ Disoriented in time or place □ Seizures, hallucinations, delirium
Lips, mouth, airway, voice	Swelling of lips, tongue, hoarse voice, stridor
Respiratory rate	<8 or >25 breaths per minute
Pulse	<45 or >130 beats per minute or irregular rhythm
Systolic blood pressure (see p.181)	<90mmHg or >160mmHg
Capillary refill test (see p.181)	>4 seconds (take care in a cold environment—it will be prolonged anyway)
Blood glucose	<3.3mmol/l (60mg/dl)
Color of skin	Very pale or yellow (jaundiced)
Size and responsiveness of pupils (see p.93)	□ Compare pupils to an unaffected team member □ Unresponsive to light stimulus
Temperature	<95°F (35°C) or >101°F (38.5°C)
Urine output	<20ml/hour (for an adult)
Diarrhea	Copious, watery, bloody

If any of these danger signs are present, seek medical advice immediately. **Urgent evacuation may be required.** Watch closely for deterioration.

3 Immediate treatment

Skin and mouth (mucosal) rashes, eruptions, blisters
□ Wash affected skin copiously with drinkable water.
□ For oral contacts, gargle and flush with drinkable water—do not swallow.
□ Give antihistamines for itching (see p.165).
□ Give topical corticosteroids for treatment of rash (see p.166).
□ Leave blisters intact as far as possible.
□ Clean raw areas with sterile fluid, and apply sterile dressing.
□ Watch for spreading infection from raw areas. Treat with antibiotics (see p.166).

Reduce absorption of toxins
Aim to implement within a few hours. However, do not put anything in the mouth or down a nasogastric (NG) tube if the casualty is sleepy or unconscious—you risk making the situation worse through aspiration.
Gastric lavage: have the casualty head down and lying on their side. Pass an NG tube (see p.200). Once certain it is in the stomach, try to suck all fluid out of the

stomach. Once empty, pass warm water down the tube (50–100ml or so) and then suck it back up. Do this until what is coming up is completely clear.
Activated charcoal: only do this with a fully conscious casualty. It is extremely dangerous if aspirated. Give 1g/kg initially, and then 1g/kg every 4 hours for several doses. Some authorities say to continue until it comes out in the stool.
Milk: regular milk for several hours post-ingestion may slow down absorption of toxins, reducing the peak effect. Only give if the casualty is fully conscious.

Nausea and vomiting
☐ Ondansetron 4mg orally (as "melts") or IV every 8 hours
☐ Prochlorperazine 12.5mg IM then oral dosing 6 hours later
☐ Cyclizine 50mg IM every 8 hours

Diarrhea
☐ Loperamide 4mg orally immediately then 2mg every episode of diarrhea (8mg max/24hrs)

Using local plants as a food source

If lost in the wilderness, a well-nourished person can survive for many days without food. The priority should be on finding clean water, without which survival, even in a temperate climate, may be less than five days. Resist the temptation to try to "live off the land," unless you are familiar with local plants and fungi.

The indigenous population, however, will have extensive knowledge about what is safe and what is poisonous; a local guide may therefore be able to help. Some common local foods require special preparation to reduce toxicity. Note that cooking does not always eliminate the toxins in fungi.

Cassava (manioc, yuca and other names) A very common source of carbohydrate in the third world, and when ground in to flour is known as tapioca. There are bitter and sweet forms, and particularly the former contains significant amounts of cyanogenic glycosides, which may release cyanide in the body. The roots should be soaked for three days and the flour soaked for at least five hours prior to cooking. Chronic poisoning leads to gradual paralysis of the legs and difficulty walking (a disease known as "konzo" in Africa).

Apples, cherries, peaches, apricots, plums and wild almonds Contain significant amounts of cyanogenic glycosides in their seeds and sometimes their leaves, so should be avoided in large quantities. Domestic almonds contain much less cyanogenic glycoside.

Indian peas (grass pea, almorta, khesari) Contain ß-N-oxalyl-L-α,ß-diaminopropionic acid (ODAP). Prolonged consumption causes weakness of the legs and wasting of the buttocks (gluteal muscles). Thorough soaking and washing, fermentation and boiling reduces the toxic effects.

Lima beans (butter beans) Contain cyanogenic glycosides. Ingesting raw or undercooked beans may cause headaches, dizziness, vertigo, confusion, weakness and chest tightness (symptoms of acute cyanide poisoning).

Kidney beans (common beans) Contain phytohemagglutinin, which, if the beans are eaten raw, causes nausea and vomiting, usually within three hours of eating, followed by diarrhea. Symptoms usually resolve in six hours without medical treatment. All beans should be boiled for at least ten minutes. Red beans produce worse symptoms than white beans.

ANIMALS AND INSECTS

Most animals will seek to escape from a direct encounter if given the chance and will only attack for defense or if they mistake a human for prey. The risk of serious injury is low but should not be ignored.

In many cases of envenomation, the insect or animal (if small or in a marine environment) will not be identified. However, it is important to recognize the symptoms and signs, know how to treat them and most importantly to know when to seek advice and evacuate. Anaphylaxis is rare but requires immediate treatment.

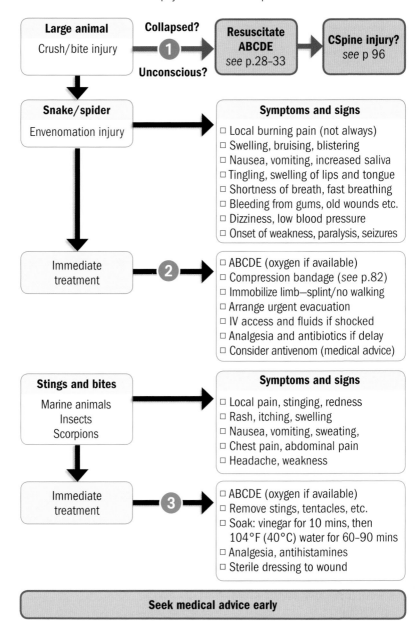

Large animal
Crush/bite injury

Collapsed?
Unconscious?

①

Resuscitate ABCDE
see p.28-33

CSpine injury?
see p 96

Snake/spider
Envenomation injury

Symptoms and signs
- Local burning pain (not always)
- Swelling, bruising, blistering
- Nausea, vomiting, increased saliva
- Tingling, swelling of lips and tongue
- Shortness of breath, fast breathing
- Bleeding from gums, old wounds etc.
- Dizziness, low blood pressure
- Onset of weakness, paralysis, seizures

Immediate treatment

②

- ABCDE (oxygen if available)
- Compression bandage (see p.82)
- Immobilize limb—splint/no walking
- Arrange urgent evacuation
- IV access and fluids if shocked
- Analgesia and antibiotics if delay
- Consider antivenom (medical advice)

Stings and bites
Marine animals
Insects
Scorpions

Symptoms and signs
- Local pain, stinging, redness
- Rash, itching, swelling
- Nausea, vomiting, sweating,
- Chest pain, abdominal pain
- Headache, weakness

Immediate treatment

③

- ABCDE (oxygen if available)
- Remove stings, tentacles, etc.
- Soak: vinegar for 10 mins, then 104°F (40°C) water for 60-90 mins
- Analgesia, antihistamines
- Sterile dressing to wound

Seek medical advice early

Anaphylaxis

Symptoms and signs	Treatment
□ General skin flushing □ Swelling of lips and eyes □ Fast pulse □ Faintness □ Wheezy chest □ Shock □ Collapse	□ ABCDE if collapsed □ Epinephrine 0.5mg IM (0.5ml of 1:1000 solution) □ Antihistamine: chlorpheniramine 10-20mg IM □ Steroid: hydrocortisone 100mg IM or IV □ IV fluids (500ml immediately) □ **Further treatment**—see p.49

Severity of envenomation

The degree of envenomation will indicate how fast you need to act.

No envenomation	Visible fang marks but no local pain/redness
Mild envenomation	Fang marks; local pain and swelling up to 10 cm in 5 hours; no systemic symptoms
Moderate envenomation	Fang marks; pain and swelling beyond 10 cm in 12 hours; bleeding from bite site; systemic symptoms —tingling, nausea and vomiting; low blood pressure
Severe envenomation	Fang marks; rapid progression of symptoms; marked swelling of extremity; bleeding from gums; shortness of breath; very low blood pressure; collapse

1 Large animal—crush or bite injury

□ **If collapsed, difficulty breathing**—*see* **p.48-49.**
□ **In severe injury, retrieve casualty from danger and treat as trauma.**
□ Stop bleeding with direct pressure (not tourniquet if possible—*see* p.88-89).
□ Clean wound with soap and water then sterile fluid (chlorhexidine, iodine).
□ Remove dead tissue, dislodged teeth, contamination.
□ Do not suture wounds—leave open and wick if necessary (*see* p.197).
□ Cover wound with sterile dressing and check daily for infection.
□ Immobilize limb, hand, foot with splint or sling (*see* p.203-5).
□ Give broad spectrum antibiotics (amoxicillin + clavulanate, doxycycline, ciprofloxacin).
□ Give analgesia.
□ Check tetanus status and availability of an antivenom.
□ In bites, check for presence of rabies in area and treat accordingly.

2 Snake/spider envenomation

□ Move casualty from danger. Do not attempt to capture or kill the snake or spider. A photograph might be useful for identification.
□ Lie casualty flat and avoid movement to slow venom absorption.
□ Remove tight clothing, jewelry before swelling starts (cut to avoid movement).
□ Apply sterile dressing then compression bandage (*see* p.82).
  - Pit viper bites do not require compression, but apply if there is any doubt.
  - DO NOT REMOVE BANDAGE until casualty is under direct medical care.

□ Immobilize casualty and with splint/slings; keep bitten part level with heart.
□ Give analgesia (not NSAIDs as they worsen bleeding) and antibiotics if signs of infection (amoxicillin + clavulanate, doxycycline, ciprofloxacin).
□ Measure blood pressure, and consider IV access and fluid.
□ Get medical advice urgently, and arrange evacuation.
□ Consider antivenom if available, but only proceed with medical advice. There is a high risk of anaphylaxis that requires urgent treatment (get IV access prior).

Applying a compression bandage

 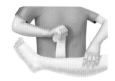

□ Using a broad, elasticated crepe bandage, start binding fingers or toes first.
□ Move up the limb toward the armpit or groin (**1**).
□ Bind tightly but not too tight to stop distal perfusion (**2**). Check distal pulses and capillary refill (*see* p.181).
□ Bind splint to arm or leg to immobilize (**3**).
□ Keep bitten part at level of heart with no movement (**4**).

❸ Stings, bites and penetrating wounds

□ Avoid getting the stings or tentacles on yourself—use gloves.
□ Soak the area in vinegar for 10 mins. This neutralizes the venom (occasionally exacerbates injury, so stop if the pain increases).
□ Cover the area with shaving cream, flour or sand/seawater paste and scrape a knife across to remove stingers—this avoids any further envenomation.
□ Remove embedded spines if possible. DO NOT remove large spines embedded in the chest, head, neck, abdomen (e.g. from a stingray)—bleeding may worsen.
□ Stop bleeding with direct pressure (not tourniquet if possible—*see* p.88-89).
□ Soak the area in very warm water for 60-90 minutes to break down venom.
□ Thoroughly wash the area, and put sterile dressings on wounds.
□ For relief of pain—ibuprofen gel and lidocaine 2% gel are effective.
□ For itching—oral antihistamine (loratidine or cetirizine).
□ For inflammation—hydrocortisone 1% cream is effective.
□ For penetrating wounds—broad spectrum antibiotics (amoxicillin + clavulanate).
□ Check tetanus status and availability of an antivenom.
□ Observe the casualty and check wounds for signs of infection, deterioration.

Prevention

Animals	Insects
□ Do not harass animals at any time	□ Use permethrin-impregnated bed nets and clothing
□ Avoid direct eye contact	□ Shake out shoes, clothing, bags
□ Store food away from living areas,	□ Use insect repellent frequently
□ Keep away from dogs/other canines	□ Wear long-sleeved shirts, pants, hats
□ Wear shoes at all times	□ Clear camp of rocks, scrub to avoid scorpions, spiders
□ Do not submerge open wounds	
□ Update tetanus vaccination	□ Avoid perfumes, deodorizers—they attract mosquitoes
□ Carry antivenom in high-risk areas	

Geographical spread of hazardous snakes, spiders and marine animals

Animal	Geographical range
Snakes	
Boomslang	Africa
Burrowing asp	Africa
Bushmaster*	S America
Carpet viper, African puff adder, horned viper	Africa, C Asia
Cat snake	Asia, Australasia
Copperhead*	N America
Coral snake	N & S America, Asia
Cobra	Africa, C & SE Asia
European adder	Europe
Krait	C and SE Asia
Mamba	Africa
Moccasin*	N America, Asia
Rattlesnake*	N & S America
Russell's viper	C & SE Asia
Brown snake, Australian copperhead, taipan, tiger snake, death adder	Australasia
Twig snake	Africa
Spiders	
Funnel-web	Australasia
Recluse	All areas except Asia
Wandering, banana	S America
Widow, redback	All areas
Water animals that sting	
Fire coral	Tropical/subtropical
Jellyfish, sea anemones	All areas
Portuguese man o'war	All areas
Water animals that jab with spines	
Catfish	Marine, estuarine, fresh water
Cone shell, sea urchins	Tropical and subtropical
Stinging fish (lionfish, scorpionfish, stonefish, needlefish, weaverfish)	Tropical and subtropical (weaverfish—temperate)
Stingray	Atlantic, Pacific, Indian Oceans; Freshwater (S America)
Water animals that bite	
Barracuda	Tropical and subtropical
Crocodile, alligator	Tropical and subtropical
Moray eel	Tropical
Sea snake	Tropical and subtropical (fresh and sea)
Shark	All areas (except polar)
Dangerous small marine animals	
Blue ringed octopus, spotted octopus, flower sea urchin	Indian/Pacific tropics
Box jellyfish	SE Asia, N Australia
Irukandji jellyfish	SE Asia, N Australia
Needlefish	Caribbean, W Africa, Japan, Indian Ocean

*From the viper subfamily Croatalinae, known as pit vipers.

SURVIVAL IN THE WILDERNESS

"Thou shalt regard Nature as thy friend, drawing thy wants from its bountiful store"—6th commandment for survivors in the bush

The ability to find water, create shelter and promote rescue are essential links in the chain of survival, and if any link is broken, survival becomes less likely.

Preparation, as always, forms a solid base to build on. Planning for unexpected events and taking sensible, necessary equipment in the form of a "survival kit" is one part of good preparation. Accumulate knowledge of how to use all possible aspects of the surrounding environment to best effect, if the expedition becomes derailed.

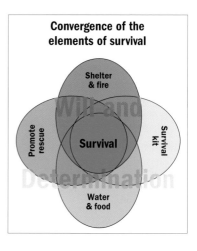

Convergence of the elements of survival

Contents of a survival kit

Rule number one is to only take a piece of kit when you know how to use it. Otherwise, it is just an encumbrance, and could have been replaced with a more useful item. Rule number two is to take one or two back-up devices for essential activities such as communication and navigation.

The survival kit should complement and reinforce the regular equipment on an expedition. It should not be "raided" during the normal course of events, and it should be reviewed regularly, particularly at points of re-supply, with any deficiencies made good. Medical content usually should be in the form of a first aid kit, which provides back-up for the main medical kit. Include emergency food.

The parameters that define the kit contents are environment (hot, cold, high altitude, jungle, marine, degree of isolation) and the number, age and fitness of expedition members. The contents should facilitate building a shelter, making and/or cleaning water, obtaining food, navigation, making a fire and communication with the outside world.

Suggested survival kit for a wilderness expedition of several days

- Emergency food
- Water container (metal)
- Water disinfection kit
- Compact cooking stove
- Matches in waterproof box, metal striker
- Cigarette lighters
- Fire lighting material (petroleum-based etc.)
- Plastic/nylon sheet or tarp 4m x 4m
- Nylon braided cord 3–30m
- Spare head torch and batteries
- Spare glasses/ sunglasses
- Fish hooks and line, thin wire for traps
- First aid kit (plus usual meds)
- Insect repellent (DEET based)
- Sunscreen and lip protection
- Multitool with blade
- Roll of duct tape and cord
- Whistle
- Signalling mirror
- Cell phone and/or satellite phone
- Personal locator beacon + GPS
- Magnetic compass and area map
- Solar charger/ Power monkey™
- Magnifying glass

Additional items for specific environments

COLD/HIGH ALTITUDE:
- Extra clothing
- Down jacket/ over pants
- Over gloves/mittens
- Goggles, face mask
- Survival bag (breathable)
- Thin foam mat (closed cell)
- Stove and extra fuel
- Extra emergency food

- Avalanche gear (shovel/probe/beacon)
- Medications for high altitude illness— see p.58-59

HOT:
- Wide-brimmed hat
- Extra sunscreen and lip protection
- Spare sunglasses
- Full length light

shirt/pants
- Equipment for making stills (see p.86)
- Steel shovel

JUNGLE/TROPICAL:
- Insect repellent, and extra medications to treat infections
- Hammock and mosquito nets
- Machete, hand saw

Shelter

Requirements
- Protection from the elements: warmth in cold climates; shade and cool in hot climates; dry in the wet
- Protection from energy loss and dehydration
- Protection from animal attack
- Psychological support, morale boost

Guide
- Small shelters are easier to build and warmer.
- Choose site that avoids risks of rock fall, avalanche, flooding, animals, bad weather.
- Use local features to aid construction—overhanging banks, caves, rock edges, fallen trees, depressions around tree trunks, overhanging branches, snow drifts.
- Construct a temporary simple shelter first if protection is required quickly for injured casualty, severe weather etc.
- If using a fire or stove inside the shelter, make a ventilation shaft. Be aware of the risks of carbon monoxide poisoning (see p.168-170).
- Avoid lying directly on snow. Use foam mat, packs, local vegetation as insulation.
- A more robust, elaborate shelter is required if a prolonged stay is anticipated (insulation, waterproofing, ventilation).

Fire

Requirements
- Warmth
- Cooking food, heating water, sterilizing
- Deterring large animals and insects
- Signalling—light and smoke

Guide
- Plan ahead and take a reliable method to light a fire, together with tinder etc.
- Don't set fire to your surrounding environment—use a fire pit and clear surrounds.
- Gather and "grade" wood—tinder, kindling, medium sticks and large logs.
- Dead wood burns better than green wood.
- Keep fuel dry if possible.
- Fires produce fumes and carbon monoxide if insufficient airflow. Use a ventilation shaft if in a shelter.
- A "heat reflector" increases the "warmth efficiency" of a fire.
- When finished, put the fire out, and make sure it's still out before leaving.

Water

Requirements (see p.72)
□ Minimum 1.5-1.8L per day for 70kg sedentary person in temperate climate
□ From reliable source or purified and disinfected (do so anyway)

Guide
□ Carry a reserve supply of water, particularly when in a vehicle (good capacity).
□ Do not :
  - Drink your own urine or anyone else's
  - Drink seawater or instil seawater into the rectum
  - Drink water from a vehicle radiator (it may contain antifreeze)
  - Ingest sea ice—it contains a high percentage of salt (upper layers less so)
  - Ingest snow to excess—it may reduce core body temperature significantly
  - Over-exert and sweat. Keep in the shade and keep cool
  - Eat too much—the process of digestion uses body water.
□ Treat all water from whatever source.
□ Never miss an opportunity to collect water. A dark plastic sheet can be used both to collect rain water, and also to melt snow/ice.
□ Observe your environment for signs of water:
  - Converging animal tracks lead to water.
  - Circling birds will often be over water.
  - Green vegetation in the desert indicates water underground.
□ Make water:
  - Melt compact snow or ice in preference to soft snow (more efficient).
  - Make a solar still to extract water from vegetation and to purify urine, radiator water, or contaminated water—see typical arrangement, below.
  - Use mashed plant matter (cacti are particularly good) to augment the output from a solar still.

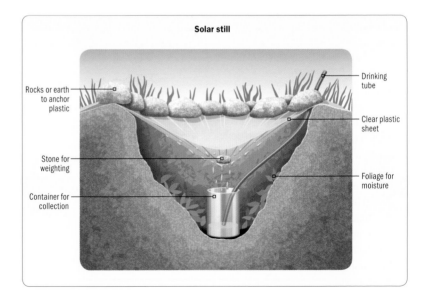

Solar still

Rocks or earth to anchor plastic

Stone for weighting

Container for collection

Drinking tube

Clear plastic sheet

Foliage for moisture

Food

Requirements
- Survival is possible even after 10–20 days without food (depending on environment, injuries, prior fitness and prior nutritional state).
- However, good nutrition increases the will and determination to survive and also increases the capacity for self-help (building, collecting/making water, signalling).

Guide
- Use emergency food sparingly.
- Observe animal behavior and eat only what they eat (reduces risk).
- Use survival kit resources to catch food (wire snares, spears, bow and arrow, fish hooks, battery light at night to attract insects and fish).
- Avoid any suspicious source of food (unknown plants, carrion etc.).
- Store any food up trees, away from camp, out of reach of bears etc.

Promoting rescue

Requirements
- Communication: cell phone, personal locator beacon, satellite phone, power supply
- Signalling: signalling mirror, whistle, signs on snow, beach etc.
- Position: rescue will be quicker if you are close to a known route, and visible.

Guide
- Leave a route plan and schedule with someone responsible (include time contingency for small mishaps).
- Always try to know where you are and which direction you are taking.
- A compass and one, preferably two, GPS devices make navigation a lot easier.
- Ensure communication devices have power. You may need high ground for a signal.
- If lost, stop. In case of poor visibility, disorientation, night time, and injury, stay put and seek/make shelter. Decide whether you can self-rescue or require rescue.
- In the case of disabling injury, decide whether the casualty can be transported. If not, send the most capable team members to get help.
- If you can self-rescue, mark your present position with something bright (and a note), and mark your way as you go. You can always return to your original position.
- In hot conditions, do not travel during the day.
- If with a crashed vehicle or aircraft, stay with it. It provides shelter, resources such as fuel, and it's usually visible from a distance.
- If you require rescue, communicate your circumstances and position electronically, if possible. Otherwise, send as SOS signal (three short, three long, three short) using a whistle or flash. Also, any signal repeated three times is a distress signal.
- Lay visual signals for searching aircraft. Letters should be a minimum of 1m high, placed high up and plainly visible. If near the sea, the beach is ideal. "V" asks for assistance. "X" asks for medical assistance. "→" indicates "travel in this direction."
- Fire at night and smoke during the day are very effective signals.
- A mirror is an effective way of "flashing" and can be seen many miles away.
- While awaiting rescue, maintain shelter and fire, and find water and food.

WOUNDS AND BLEEDING

Accidents that cause wounds and bleeding happen often on expeditions. They should be treated quickly and effectively to avoid complications. The expedition leader and medic should know how best to minimize blood loss, preventing an injury from becoming a serious threat. Follow a structured approach to avoid complications and encourage healing.

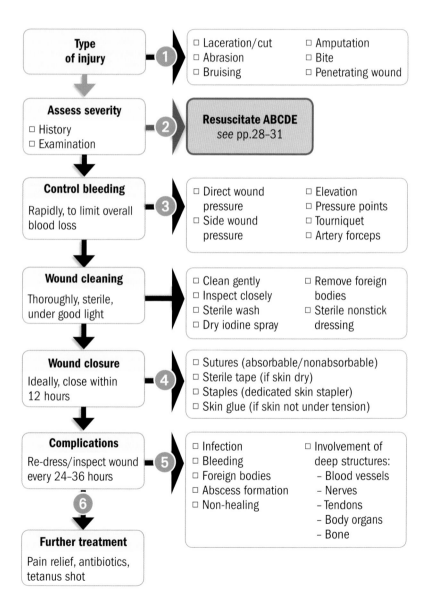

Type of injury ➊
- Laceration/cut
- Abrasion
- Bruising
- Amputation
- Bite
- Penetrating wound

Assess severity ➋
- History
- Examination

Resuscitate ABCDE
see pp.28–31

Control bleeding
Rapidly, to limit overall blood loss ➌
- Direct wound pressure
- Side wound pressure
- Elevation
- Pressure points
- Tourniquet
- Artery forceps

Wound cleaning
Thoroughly, sterile, under good light
- Clean gently
- Inspect closely
- Sterile wash
- Dry iodine spray
- Remove foreign bodies
- Sterile nonstick dressing

Wound closure
Ideally, close within 12 hours ➍
- Sutures (absorbable/nonabsorbable)
- Sterile tape (if skin dry)
- Staples (dedicated skin stapler)
- Skin glue (if skin not under tension)

Complications
Re-dress/inspect wound every 24–36 hours ➎
- Infection
- Bleeding
- Foreign bodies
- Abscess formation
- Non-healing
- Involvement of deep structures:
  - Blood vessels
  - Nerves
  - Tendons
  - Body organs
  - Bone

➏

Further treatment
Pain relief, antibiotics, tetanus shot

① Type of injury

Cuts and lacerations Cuts are made by sharp objects. They are usually clean-edged and heal well. Lacerations are made by blunt objects. They are more ragged, more difficult to repair, and more likely to become infected. If a wound is close to a bony fracture, treat it as a compound fracture (*see* p.206).

Abrasion In the event of a small abrasion, or graze, simply clean the affected area. Severe abrasions may cause significant tissue loss and necessitate eventual surgery. Clean major abrasions thoroughly to avoid "tattooing" (discolored scarring) and give antibiotics if the casualty has lost a lot of tissue.

Bruising Bruises (hematomas) are usually thought of as minor, but occasionally when blood collects in the tissues it becomes infected and causes an abscess that needs to be drained. Watch for signs of infection.

Amputations The accidental severing, or traumatic amputation, of a finger or toe is not uncommon, particularly on boats. Evacuate the casualty as soon as possible and keep the digit cool but not frozen. Seek medical advice as soon as possible. The severing of an arm or leg is a threat to life and a medical emergency.

Bites Bites, both human and animal, contain a lot of bacteria and often become infected. Clean any bites very thoroughly and administer antibiotics.

Penetrating wounds Wounds that pierce the skin and pass into tissue are difficult to assess. Organs, bone, tendons, nerves or blood vessels may have been affected, so the casualty should be closely observed. Seek medical advice early.

② Assess severity

History The mechanism of injury may give an idea about extent and severity.

Important points in the history

- How did the accident happen? (knife, glass, energy involved)
- When and where did it happen?
- Was the casualty crushed at all?
- Is there risk of contamination?
- Who else was involved?
- Date of last tetanus vaccination?

Examination Carry out the examination in a well-lit, secure place where you can take your time. Complete examination of a penetrating wound is impossible in the wilderness, but try to be thorough, inspecting as much of the wound as you can for contamination. Use local anesthetic (*see* pp.198–99).

Important points in the examination

- Size and shape of wound
- Contamination and foreign bodies
- Presence of pulse beyond injury
- Signs of nerve damage:
  - Sensation
  - Movement
- Signs of infection:
  - Redness around the wound
  - Painful swelling
  - Swollen lymph nodes in groin, armpit
  - Lymphangitis: red streaks spreading up the arm or leg

---

③ Control bleeding

- Limit or stop bleeding as quickly as possible.
- Control bleeding from a vein by raising the limb above the heart.
- Bleeding from an artery may spurt with the pulse. Apply direct pressure to the wound or pressure on each side if direct pressure is too painful.
- Clamp an obviously spurting vessel with artery clamps and tie off with a suture.
- Use pressure points (in the armpit or groin for arm/leg wounds), tourniquets or artery forceps only if direct pressure does not work; blood flow to the extremity of the limb may be dangerously reduced by these methods, but they may become necessary.

④ Wound closure (see p.88)

- Ideally, wounds should be closed within 12–24 hours after thorough cleaning.
- If it is impossible to clean the wound, it may be better left open until it can be cleaned surgically
- Wound closure is an effective way of reducing blood loss.
- Absorbable sutures are usually used to close layers of tissue below the skin. Use nonabsorbable sutures for the skin.
- Sterile adhesive skin tape is effective for small wounds, if the skin is dry.
- Skin staples from a dedicated skin stapler are rapid and good for wet skin.
- Tissue adhesive (skin glue) is fast but useless if the skin is damp or under tension.
- Healing will be improved, especially of large wounds, if the limb is immobilized to prevent stretching of the skin repair. The casualty should rest as much as possible.

⑤ Complications

- Wounds often become infected. Inspect the area every 24–36 hours and apply a fresh sterile dressing. Treat any suspected infection with broad-spectrum antibiotics immediately.
- Infection may cause bleeding to start again a few days after the accident. Thoroughly clean infected tissue under local anesthetic (may be only partially effective). Seek medical advice.
- Foreign bodies (dirt, grit, etc.) may cause infection or discolored scarring if they are not removed immediately.
- Damage to structures below the skin may cause a wide variety of complications. If there is ongoing pain, loss of movement or sensation, or bleeding, seek medical advice regarding further treatment, particularly for penetrating wounds.

⑥ Further treatment

- Antibiotics are always indicated for:
  - Heavily contaminated wounds
  - Any form of bite
  - Fractures where the bone comes through the skin
  - Traumatic amputation
  - Wounds that become infected
- Pain relief is essential and should be given as soon as possible.
- Local anesthetic injection (infiltration) around wounds will help examination and repair (see pp.198–99).
- **Check that the person's tetanus vaccination is up to date.**

HEAD INJURIES

It is not uncommon for expedition members to sustain minor head injuries. In most cases they will recover quickly and suffer no lasting damage. Serious head injuries occur less often but may threaten life. These cases call for immediate evacuation.

The priorities in treating a head injury are to maintain blood pressure and oxygenation and prevent complications. Effective action will reduce the risk of deterioration.

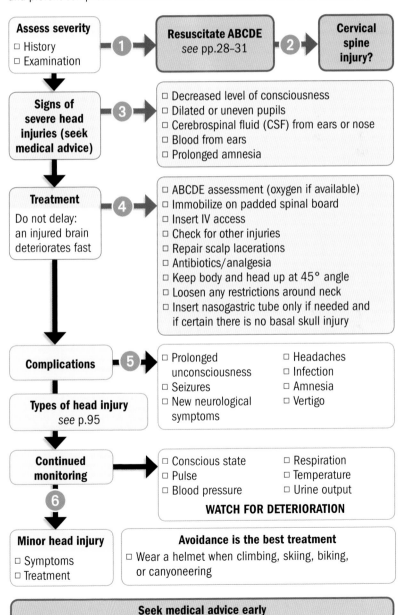

Assess severity
- History
- Examination

1 → **Resuscitate ABCDE** *see pp.28–31* **2** → **Cervical spine injury?**

Signs of severe head injuries (seek medical advice) **3** →
- Decreased level of consciousness
- Dilated or uneven pupils
- Cerebrospinal fluid (CSF) from ears or nose
- Blood from ears
- Prolonged amnesia

Treatment
Do not delay: an injured brain deteriorates fast **4** →
- ABCDE assessment (oxygen if available)
- Immobilize on padded spinal board
- Insert IV access
- Check for other injuries
- Repair scalp lacerations
- Antibiotics/analgesia
- Keep body and head up at 45° angle
- Loosen any restrictions around neck
- Insert nasogastric tube only if needed and if certain there is no basal skull injury

Complications **5** →
- Prolonged unconsciousness
- Seizures
- New neurological symptoms
- Headaches
- Infection
- Amnesia
- Vertigo

Types of head injury *see p.95*

Continued monitoring →
- Conscious state
- Pulse
- Blood pressure
- Respiration
- Temperature
- Urine output

WATCH FOR DETERIORATION

6

Minor head injury
- Symptoms
- Treatment

Avoidance is the best treatment
- Wear a helmet when climbing, skiing, biking, or canyoneering

Seek medical advice early

① History and examination

- ABCDE assessment (*see* pp. 30–33) takes priority over everything else.
- Take particular care of the neck (*see* below).
- A conscious casualty is reassuring but may deteriorate later.
- Get as much information as possible from other team members.

Important points in the history

- How did the accident happen?
- Was there loss of consciousness? For how long?
- Does the casualty have loss of memory (amnesia) and for how long?
- Has the casualty been sick, or does he or she feel sick?
- Does the casualty have a headache?

Important points in the examination

- Level of consciousness (*see* below)
- Size and reactivity of pupils (*see* below)
- Weakness or paralysis of face or limbs
- Heart rate, blood pressure, respiratory rate
- Twitching, seizures

---

② Cervical spine (neck) injury

Spinal injuries are common with head injuries. The bones of the neck may be broken and be unstable, but the spinal cord may still be intact. If in doubt, immobilize the cervical spine (*see* pp.178–79).

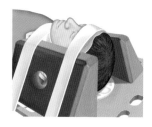

Cervical spine immobilization

③ Signs of severe head injury

Level of consciousness In general, the worse the conscious level, the worse the head injury. A casualty may initially appear to be conscious after an injury but may deteriorate rapidly. Therefore, monitor conscious level frequently.

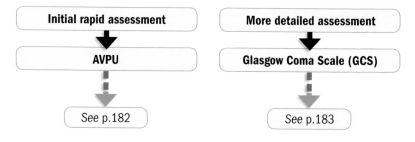

Initial rapid assessment	More detailed assessment
↓	↓
AVPU	**Glasgow Coma Scale (GCS)**
↓	↓
See p.182	See p.183

If the casualty is less than "alert" on the AVPU scale, assess using GCS. Reassess every 15 minutes for at least the first few hours.

- GCS score 9–12: possible significant head injury
- GCS score <8: serious head injury
- Reduction in GCS score of 2 or more: serious deterioration

Seek medical advice early

Dilated or uneven pupils Pupils should normally be equal and reactive to light. A head injury may cause the pupils to be: unequal in size; unreactive to light; dilated and unreactive.

Pupil size	Pupil response to light	Likely cause
Both pupils equally dilated	Responsive equally	Fear, alcohol, drugs such as cocaine
Both pupils equally constricted	Responsive equally	Bright light, drugs such as opiates or benzodiazepines
Pupils uneven	Larger pupil unresponsive	Head injury, eye injury or direct drug contamination (such as with scopolamine)
Both pupils dilated	Both pupils unresponsive	Severe injury to head, death

Cerebrospinal fluid (CSF) or blood from the ears CSF is clear and similar in appearance to tears or saliva. This is important to remember if you see clear fluid around the head. Blood in the ears may have originated inside the head, but could also have run into the ears from wounds on the scalp or face. If you are uncertain, assume clear fluid is CSF, and assume that fluid in the ears has come from inside the head until proven otherwise.

Prolonged post-traumatic amnesia (PTA) It is quite common for casualties to experience a short period of memory loss following head injury. A period of amnesia lasting longer than 30 minutes indicates a significant head injury.

④ Treatment

A casualty with a suspected head injury should be evacuated as soon as possible.
Treatment in the wilderness is aimed at preventing complications. Once the casualty has been assessed for ABCDE, given oxygen if available, and immobilized on a padded, rigid board to protect potential spinal fractures and prevent pressure sores, it is important to look for other injuries (the secondary survey–*see* pp.32-33).
A casualty who has received a head injury and who is also in shock is very likely to have another injury.
☐ Scalp lacerations bleed heavily, and a lot of blood may be lost in a short time. Repair them as quickly as possible, by suturing, stapling or gluing.
☐ IV fluids may be required to restore blood pressure to normal.
☐ The casualty should be kept head–up if possible, which can be achieved by tilting the rigid board. If there are any tight restrictions around the neck, such as a dry-suit seal, these should be removed. These maneuvers help to reduce the pressure in the brain.
☐ DO NOT put in a nasogastric tube if there are signs of a basal skull fracture (black eyes, blood, or CSF from ears or nose). In these cases there is a danger that the tube may end up in the brain.
☐ Avoid giving morphine to head injured casualties. Regular acetaminophen and codeine may be used and should not reduce the conscious level.
☐ If there is suspicion of a skull fracture, give antibiotics.

⑤ Complications

Medical help should have been sought by this stage and MUST be sought if there are any signs of complications. Any sign of deterioration in the casualty's conscious level or new signs of paralysis of the face or one side of the body are ominous and the casualty must be evacuated urgently. Managing an unconscious casualty in the wilderness for a prolonged period is a complex and difficult task. The issues involved are described on pp.34-36.

Seizures Seizures are common after relatively minor head injuries, and should stop by themselves after a minute or so. Recurrent, prolonged seizures (seizures that last longer than 1-2 minutes) are much more concerning and should be treated (*see* p.38).

Signs of infection Temperature, flushing or signs of meningism (*see* p.133), such as photophobia (intolerance of bright light), stiffness in the neck and headache, are very serious because they may indicate an infection. Administer IV broad-spectrum antibiotics.

Vertigo The whirling sensations associated with vertigo are common following a head injury, and these symptoms may be treated using either prochlorperazine or cyclizine.

Headaches Use nonsedating painkillers if possible. Worsening of a headache may indicate worsening of the head injury, so seek medical advice.

⑥ Minor head injuries

Symptoms	☐ Dizziness ☐ Vomiting (no more than 3 times) ☐ Headache ☐ Tiredness ☐ Difficulty concentrating
Treatment	☐ Nonsedating painkillers for headache. ☐ Prochlorperazine or cyclizine for dizziness/nausea. ☐ Rest for a few days as necessary, avoiding strenuous activities. ☐ Watch for deterioration in conscious level or vital signs.
Outlook	Symptoms should last only a few days at most. Seek medical advice if they persist longer than this.

Types of head injuries

Closed Closed head injuries are the most common type. There is no fracture (or only minor fracture) of the skull, and the brain is not exposed. These injuries are usually caused by a blunt blow to the head, such as collision with the ground or a tree trunk.

Open Less common than closed injuries, open injuries are usually more serious. The brain is exposed, which may be obvious to the untrained eye, but will sometimes be difficult to assess in cases of basal skull fracture. Open head injuries are usually caused by sharp objects or small, blunt objects, such as rocks, and carry a high risk of infection. There are three types of open head injury:

☐ Penetrating: when a sharp object, such as a spear, goes through the skull and into the brain.
☐ Compound depressed skull fracture: caused by collision with a small, solid object such as a rock. A piece of the skull is pushed into the brain.
☐ Basal skull fracture: a type of fracture running across the base of the skull and opening up a communication between the inside of the casualty's skull and the tubes of the ears or nose.

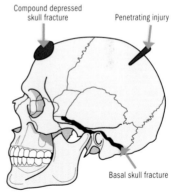

Compound depressed skull fracture

Penetrating injury

Basal skull fracture

Open head injuries

Primary injury This term refers to the direct result of the blow to the head. The primary injury could involve skull fracture, damage to the brain tissue itself, or bleeding in the brain.

Secondary injury If, after a primary injury, the brain deteriorates due to lack of blood flow or oxygen, it is known as secondary injury. In an expedition situation, resources may be limited, but a few simple actions, such as establishing an airway and immobilizing the neck, may reduce the severity of secondary injury.

NECK AND SPINAL INJURIES

Back strains and sprains are common on expeditions, especially in people who are not accustomed to physical exertion. Very occasionally, however, an injury that looks minor turns out to be very serious. If you are in any doubt, immobilize the casualty and seek medical advice. Spinal cord damage is grave and often permanent, so make sure you protect the injured or unstable spine before you move the casualty.

High-energy accidents, such as falling from a height, cause more severe injuries. Keep in mind that intoxication and visible injuries such as broken limbs and open wounds can sometimes divert attention from a spinal injury.

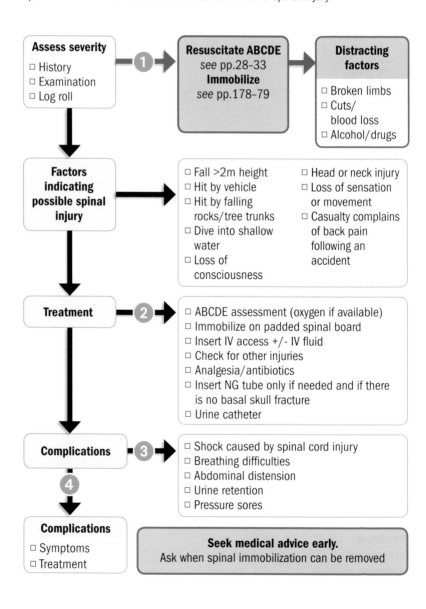

Assess severity
- □ History
- □ Examination
- □ Log roll

1 **Resuscitate ABCDE**
see pp.28–33
Immobilize
see pp.178–79

Distracting factors
- □ Broken limbs
- □ Cuts/ blood loss
- □ Alcohol/drugs

Factors indicating possible spinal injury
- □ Fall >2m height
- □ Hit by vehicle
- □ Hit by falling rocks/tree trunks
- □ Dive into shallow water
- □ Loss of consciousness
- □ Head or neck injury
- □ Loss of sensation or movement
- □ Casualty complains of back pain following an accident

Treatment **2**
- □ ABCDE assessment (oxygen if available)
- □ Immobilize on padded spinal board
- □ Insert IV access +/- IV fluid
- □ Check for other injuries
- □ Analgesia/antibiotics
- □ Insert NG tube only if needed and if there is no basal skull fracture
- □ Urine catheter

Complications **3**
- □ Shock caused by spinal cord injury
- □ Breathing difficulties
- □ Abdominal distension
- □ Urine retention
- □ Pressure sores

4

Complications
- □ Symptoms
- □ Treatment

Seek medical advice early.
Ask when spinal immobilization can be removed

❶ History and examination

Parts of the spine

Cervical vertebrae ——
(cervical spine)

Thoracic vertebrae ——

Lumbar vertebrae ——

Sacrum ——

Coccyx ——

☐ ABCDE assessment (*see* pp.28–31) takes priority over everything else.
☐ Anyone with a head injury may well have a spinal injury as well.
☐ A proper examination for possible neck and spinal injuries will require a log roll (*see* p.177), which requires four people to turn the casualty and one to examine the back.

Important points in the history

☐ How did the accident happen?
☐ Where is the pain?
☐ Are there any symptoms of nerve damage? – Numbness
       – Pins and needles
       – Loss of movement
☐ Any previous history of back pain or injuries?

Important points in the examination

Look Obvious injuries to head, neck, spine; swelling, bruising
Feel Tenderness, steps in spine, can the casualty feel touch and pain?
Move Can casualty move body and limbs? If neck injured, do not move it
Document Tone, power, sensation for all limbs and the main body

❷ Treatment

A casualty with a suspected spinal injury must be evacuated as soon as possible.
Immobilization (*see* pp.178–79) The whole body must be immobilized as effectively as possible using a semi-rigid collar and a padded board.
IV access and fluid Casualty may have low blood pressure and need IV fluid.
Nasogastric (NG) tube, urinary catheter (*see* pp.200–201) An immobilized casualty may be kept hydrated by an NG tube and will need a urinary catheter.
Analgesia, antibiotics Pain relief to settle the casualty; antibiotics for an open wound.

❸ Complications

☐ Spinal cord damage can cause blood vessels to relax, leading to low blood pressure and shock. Seek medical advice for guidance on fluid replacement.
☐ Breathing difficulties may result from spinal cord injuries located high in the chest or in the neck. This is an ominous problem. Administer oxygen if available and follow ABC assessment if the casualty stops breathing (*see* p.28).
☐ The stomach may stop working, and the casualty may vomit. Insert an NG tube and suck out the contents to reduce the risk (*see* p.200), then attach a collection bag.

❹ Minor back injuries

Symptoms A minor back injury will cause localized pain that is worse on straining or coughing. Pain may extend down the leg (sciatica) and posture may be abnormal.
Treatments Administer pain relief to allow mobilization, reducing stiffness. If the casualty has sciatica, advise rest. Care should be taken with the posture during vigorous activities such as chopping wood and carrying loads.

FACIAL INJURIES

Facial injuries look appalling, but once the blood is cleaned up, they often turn out to be minor. Be aware of cosmetic issues when treating wounds to the face.

Fractures may be difficult to detect. The first thing to consider in facial fractures is possible damage to the airway, which poses a serious threat to life; take steps to minimize this threat. Remember that swelling may compromise breathing hours after the initial injury. Head and neck injuries often accompany injuries to the face, so assess the casualty systematically using the ABCDE approach.

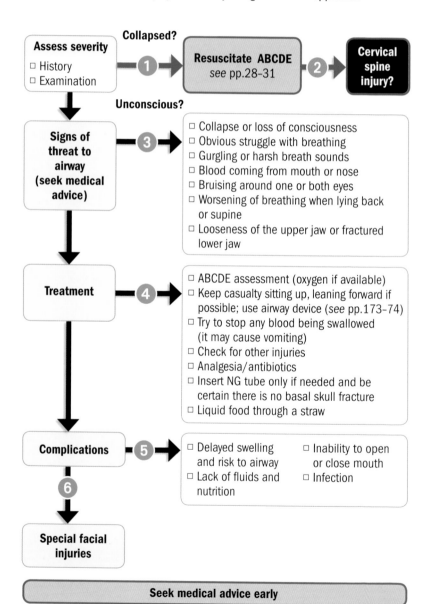

Assess severity
- □ History
- □ Examination

Collapsed?
1

Resuscitate ABCDE
see pp.28–31
2

Cervical spine injury?

Unconscious?

Signs of threat to airway (seek medical advice)
3
- □ Collapse or loss of consciousness
- □ Obvious struggle with breathing
- □ Gurgling or harsh breath sounds
- □ Blood coming from mouth or nose
- □ Bruising around one or both eyes
- □ Worsening of breathing when lying back or supine
- □ Looseness of the upper jaw or fractured lower jaw

Treatment
4
- □ ABCDE assessment (oxygen if available)
- □ Keep casualty sitting up, leaning forward if possible; use airway device (*see pp.173–74*)
- □ Try to stop any blood being swallowed (it may cause vomiting)
- □ Check for other injuries
- □ Analgesia/antibiotics
- □ Insert NG tube only if needed and be certain there is no basal skull fracture
- □ Liquid food through a straw

Complications
5
- □ Delayed swelling and risk to airway
- □ Lack of fluids and nutrition
- □ Inability to open or close mouth
- □ Infection

6

Special facial injuries

Seek medical advice early

1 History and examination

☐ Be aware that anyone with a facial injury may well have sustained additional injuries, particularly to the head and neck.

☐ It might be difficult to find out exactly what happened from the casualty who has a facial injury, so collect as much information as you can from witnesses.

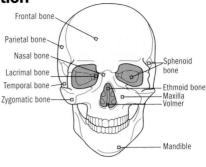

Frontal bone
Parietal bone
Nasal bone
Lacrimal bone
Temporal bone
Zygomatic bone
Sphenoid bone
Ethmoid bone
Maxilla
Volmer
Mandible

Bones of the face

Important points in the history	**Important points in the examination**
☐ How did the accident happen? ☐ Was there any loss of consciousness? For how long? ☐ Any difficulty breathing? ☐ Any problems with vision (double vision, for example)?	**Look** Obvious injuries to face, deformed nose, swelling, blood **Feel** Tenderness over cheeks, jaw, steps in bone edges, crepitus **Move** Ask casualty to open and close mouth. Do the teeth line up? Is the upper jaw loose?

---

2 Cervical spine (neck) injury

Spinal injuries commonly accompany head injuries. Keep in mind that the bones of the neck may be broken and unstable, but the spinal cord may still be intact. If you are in any doubt at all about the nature of the injury, immobilize the cervical spine (see pp.178–79).

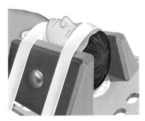

Cervical spine immobilization

3 Signs of threat to airway

When a bone is broken in the middle of the face or jaw (mandible), the fractured piece of face or jaw bone may fall back into the airway and partially or entirely block it. It is crucial to recognize the signs of an obstructed airway.

☐ The casualty may be struggling and making harsh or gurgling sounds when breathing in.

☐ Pain, swelling, bilateral black eyes and blood from the mouth may also be present and are consistent with facial fractures.

☐ If the casualty is conscious, they will be able to describe their difficulties with breathing and whether sitting up and leaning forward eases them. Being upright and leaning forward helps to clear the airway by allowing the broken part of the face or jaw to "hang forward," clearing the airway.

☐ A fracture through the mid-part of the face (the maxilla), above the upper jaw, may make the upper jaw "loose." Test this by holding the gums above the front teeth firmly with the fingers and trying gently to move the upper jaw in and out. Only do this once, as repetitions will cause pain, bleeding and further swelling.

④ Immediate treatment

☐ A casualty with a suspected facial fracture should be evacuated as soon as possible.
☐ If the casualty is conscious but having difficulty breathing, try to keep them sitting up and leaning forward.
☐ Lie unconscious casualties in the recovery position if you are sure there are no spine injuries (see pp.176–77).
☐ An airway adjunct, such as a Guedel airway, may be needed (see p.173), but insert very gently. Do not insert a nasopharyngeal airway unless absolutely certain there is no basal-skull or mid-face fracture.
☐ Either drain blood from the mouth in the recovery position or use a suction device if available. Blood in the stomach is a strong stimulus for vomiting. Any vomit may end up in the lungs.
☐ Use nonsedating painkillers—acetaminophen, nonsteroidal anti-inflammatory drugs (NSAIDs). NSAIDs may reduce swelling.
☐ Insert a nasogastric (NG) tube only if really needed, and then only if you are absolutely sure there is no basal-skull or mid-face fracture.
☐ Swallowing or chewing may be painful and difficult. It may be impossible to close the mouth. Liquid food through an NG tube or straw may be required.
☐ Use antibiotics for lacerations, continual blood in the mouth or a temperature.

⑤ Complications

☐ Swelling may get worse for a few days after the injury. Get medical advice if there is any doubt regarding the airway and arrange evacuation.
☐ If oral fluid intake is inadequate, rehydrate by another route (see pp.184).
☐ Fractures or dislocations of the jaw or cheek bones may prevent the mouth from opening or closing. A mouth which is jammed open is painful and potentially dangerous. Get medical advice and evacuate as soon as possible.
☐ Infection is a considerable risk, because fractures that run into the mouth, airway or sinuses cannot be diagnosed in the wilderness. Treat any suspected facial fractures with antibiotics until the casualty can be evacuated.

⑥ Specific facial injuries

Lacerations of the face and lips
Facial lacerations bleed heavily and look frightening before they are cleaned up. Take care when suturing, using sterile tape, or gluing, to avoid cosmetic damage. If the lips have been lacerated, realign the lip edges as accurately as possible during suturing. Administer a local anesthetic before cleaning the wound (see pp.198–99). Use interrupted sutures with the finest thread possible and give antibiotics for large or dirty wounds (see p.192–93).

Tongue injuries
If the casualty has suffered a blow to the face, the teeth may have lacerated the tongue. If there is blood in the mouth, examine the tongue carefully. If there is a serious injury, seek medical advice and keep the casualty sitting up to reduce swelling that may threaten the airway.

Fractured nose

If the nose is broken there will be a lot of blood. Stop the bleeding by squeezing the soft part of the nose firmly, and seek medical advice. It might be necessary to pack the nose with a gauze strip soaked in epinephrine or petroleum jelly. If the nose is bent, realign it immediately, if the casualty allows, before swelling occurs. Use a firm movement. If there is a tense collection of blood in the midline of the nose, drain it carefully under local anesthesia, as this may lead to tissue death if left untreated.

Fractures of the cheek bone

Symptoms and signs:

- □ A black eye/double vision
- □ Possible pain in the eye
- □ Difficulty opening mouth/chewing
- □ "Step" on lower ridge of eye socket.

Analgesia and a soft diet will reduce the discomfort caused by fractures of the cheek bone. Arrange to evacuate the casualty as soon as possible.

Fractures of the mid-face

A large amount of force is required to cause such a fracture, so other injuries are likely. Seek medical advice urgently and arrange for evacuation as soon as possible. Symptoms and signs:

- □ Difficulty with the airway
- □ Bilateral black eyes
- □ A loose upper jaw and breathing
- □ Difficulty in opening the mouth.

Assess and support the airway. This may be very difficult if the casualty is unconscious and may prove impossible without specialist equipment and immediate skilled help. Do the best you can. Other supportive treatments are outlined on pp.34–36.

Dislocated mandible

A blow to the jaw or opening the mouth very wide—during a yawn, for example—can cause dislocation of the jaw, making it impossible to close the mouth. If the jaw is twisted off to one side, only one of the joints is dislocated. The dislocation should be reduced as soon as possible. Seek medical advice. You may need to sedate the casualty to restore the jaw to the correct position.

Fractured mandible

A reasonable amount of force is required to fracture the mandible, and severe fractures may be life-threatening. Seek medical advice urgently and evacuate.

Symptoms and signs:

- □ Difficulty with airway and breathing
- □ Difficulty opening the mouth
- □ Obvious deformity of jaw line
- □ Swelling along jaw and up side of head
- □ "Step" in the teeth of the lower jaw.

Barton bandage
A Barton bandage passes around the head three times, as shown above, and is secured at the top.

Assess and support the airway as effectively as possible, though this may be very difficult, as with a mid-face fracture. The mandible can be immobilized by wiring the teeth of the lower jaw to the teeth of the upper jaw, but this requires skill and an extremely brave patient. A Barton bandage (see above) is less invasive and easier than wiring. You may need to cut the bandage off quickly if the patient vomits.

EYE INJURIES

The eyeball is relatively well protected—only about a fifth of the eyeball surface is exposed. For this reason, direct eye injuries are uncommon. When they do occur, however, eye injuries are often serious and may threaten sight. Injuries to the mid-face and cheek bone may be associated with eye injuries.

People who wear glasses can lessen the likelihood of injuries caused by shattered glass by using plastic lenses. Contact lenses can cause problems in conditions of extreme cold, heat and wind. For other eye problems, *see* pp.134–137

History

- If eye is injured, how and when?
- Duration of symptoms?
- Any history of foreign bodies in the eye?
- Painful or painless eye?
- Previous eye/vision problems
- Eye surgery in the past (cataract/laser)?
- Contact lenses or glasses?
- Diabetes or glaucoma?

Examination

This needs to be done in a safe, enclosed area. The area should be well lit, with a headlamp if necessary, and the casualty should be provided with painkillers.

Look

- Obvious bruising, swelling, lacerations
- Foreign bodies under lids or inside the eye
- Pupil size and reaction to light
- Reddened sclera
- Tears streaming from the eye
- Blood inside the eye. You may see blood in front of the iris
- Examine the cornea using magnifying glass and fluorescein eye drops—these glow in bright light, showing up abrasions. Put local anesthetic (tetracaine) drops in the eye first
- Look inside eyelids: gently pull lower lid down; turn back upper lid (*see* opposite).
- Compare one side with the other

Feel

- Bony steps around the edge of the eye socket (orbit)
- Firmness of the eyeball (gently) to get an idea of intraocular pressure

Move

- Ask casualty to look at your finger held about 30cm away
- Move the finger up and down and from side to side slowly, keeping the head still
- Ask about double vision, and watch eye movements closely
- Document any pain

Visual Acuity

- Ask the casualty whether their visual acuity is normal
- Test vision by reading small text from a book at normal distance

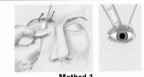 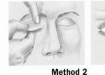

| Method 1 | Method 2 |

Examine under the upper lid, using either a cotton swab (Method 1) or a finger (Method 2) to roll back the lid.

Immediate treatment

Seek medical advice for any injuries that affect eyesight, for penetrating injuries, for chemical burns or if you are worried. Assess for other facial injuries (*see* p.98).

Pain relief

Orally   Other injuries may have occurred and the casualty will need to be comfortable to allow examination.

To the eye   Tetracaine (0.5%) local anesthetic eye drops, a few drops inside each lower lid. The local anesthetic action will last up to an hour or so. Pad the eye to protect it after examination.

Antibiotics If in doubt, apply antibiotic drops or ointment: drops are easier to use; ointment lasts longer and lubricates the eye nicely, but blurs the vision. Chloramphenicol is the usual broad-spectrum antibiotic used for the eyes. For penetrating injuries and if there is blood or foreign bodies in the eye, use oral antibiotics as well.

Eye pads Padding a painful eye will make the casualty more comfortable. Avoid applying more pressure than is necessary and do not pad both eyes at the same time unless you have to. Ensure the eyelids are shut, particularly if the eye is anesthetized; padding may scratch an eye that is not completely closed.

Foreign bodies Remove any visible foreign bodies immediately by flushing the eye with sterile saline or water, or by gently using a cotton swab.

Chemicals Flush with plenty of sterile water or saline as soon as possible after the accident, using a plastic bag with a small hole in it. Continue for at least 10 minutes or, if the chemical was an alkali, for at least 30 minutes. Do not contaminate an injured eye.

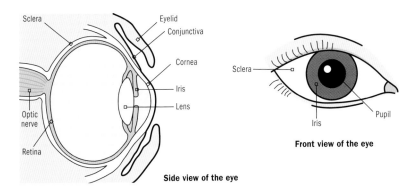

Side view of the eye

Front view of the eye

Specific eye problems

Eyelid laceration
□ This is a serious injury, often accompanied by other injures to the eye itself.
□ If the eye is left exposed, corneal damage and infection are more likely to occur.
□ Seek medical advice regarding repair.

Symptoms and signs	Treatment
□ Examine eye after local anesthetic drops □ Look carefully for other injuries, particularly if high energy involved □ Look for foreign bodies in the eye and eyelid □ Take particular care if the eyelid margin is lacerated	□ Apply firm but gentle pressure to stop bleeding □ Remove foreign bodies □ Antibiotic ointment or drops and oral broad-spectrum antibiotics to prevent orbital cellulitis/infection □ Get medical advice if you plan to attempt a repair yourself □ Pad the eye and use artificial tears if the cornea is left exposed

Corneal abrasion
Corneal abrasion is caused by a foreign body on the surface of the eye, an object hitting the open eye or lack of care with an anesthetized eye.

Symptoms and signs	Treatment
□ Painful eye □ Feels like a foreign body in the eye □ Abrasion may be seen in a magnifying glass, with the help of fluorescein staining (see p.135)	□ Flush the eye to remove any foreign bodies that remain □ Use local anesthetic drops for pain □ Administer oral pain relief if there is an accompanying headache □ Use antibiotic ointment or drops to lubricate and soothe the abrasion □ Pad the eye if particularly painful

Foreign body
The object may be under the eyelids or may even have penetrated the eyeball itself (see penetrating eye injury, below).

Symptoms and signs	Treatment
□ Mechanism of injury? □ Examine eye after local anesthetic and fluorescein drops (see p.135) □ Examine under the upper and lower eyelids (see pp.102–103) □ The eye will produce a lot of tears	□ Pain relief with local anesthetic eyedrops □ If obvious, remove foreign body with (clean) finger or cotton swab □ Flush eye with sterile water or saline. Use a clean plastic bag with a small hole in it if no syringe is available. Boil water and cool if nothing else is available □ Antibiotic ointment or drops to soothe and lubricate the eye

Chemical burn
□ Burns with alkali chemicals are generally worse than those with acids.
□ Medical advice is required for all chemical burns as soon as possible.
□ Identify which chemical was involved (for example, battery acid).

Symptoms and signs	Treatment
□ Red, painful eye □ Look for chemical burn to surrounding face □ Eyesight might be blurred □ One or both eyes may be involved	□ Start flushing eye immediately before chemical penetrates eye □ Use the cleanest water/saline available urgently (sterile preferably) □ Flush for at least 30 minutes—avoid contaminating the other eye □ Antibiotic ointment for lubrication and comfort (also use artificial tears) □ Local anesthetic drops if very painful

Nonpenetrating eye injury
□ A blunt blow to the face that may cause other facial injuries.
□ Weakest point of the orbit is the floor (below the eye), and this may "blow out" into the space (sinus) below.

Symptoms and signs	Treatment
□ Mechanism of injury? □ Black eye, swelling, bruising □ Pain on eye movement □ Injury to eye itself □ An eyeball that looks sunken □ Compare with the other side □ Assess for other injuries	□ Thoroughly examine eye before swelling prevents eye opening □ Treat other injuries □ Consider local anesthetic drops/antibiotic drops to eye if painful □ Pad/cover the eye if double vision causing distress □ Consider ice pack for swelling/bruising

Penetrating eye injury
□ This may be obvious, but might be difficult to see if small objects enter through the cornea—any hole closes quickly.
□ The energy involved in the accident is important; high-speed metal fragments are more likely to penetrate the eyeball.
□ Seek medical advice immediately, as eyesight may be threatened.

Symptoms and signs	Treatment
□ Mechanism of injury? □ Painful red eye □ Irregular pupil □ Decreased vision □ Visible foreign body in/behind cornea □ Laceration of cornea/sclera □ Soft eye to gentle pressure □ Leakage of eye contents	□ Do not remove object impaled in eye □ Guard against impaled object being pushed further in □ Antibiotic ointment or drops □ Local anesthetic drops □ Oral broad-spectrum antibiotics □ Pad over eye, with shield to prevent impaled object moving □ Seek medical advice immediately

CHEST INJURIES

"Blunt" chest injuries are usually caused by falls or collisions with vehicles. "Penetrating" chest injuries, in which a sharp object enters the chest, are rare but usually more serious.

In the wilderness, it will not be possible to distinguish between severe bruising of the chest wall and fractured ribs. Both injuries impair the casualty's ability to function and and both are treated in the same way. However, the major concern with any chest injury is damage to the heart or lungs. Any pre-existing conditions of the lungs or heart disease will complicate the situation.

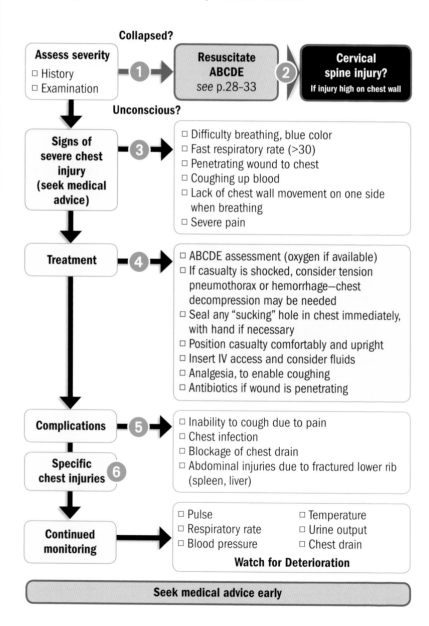

Assess severity
- History
- Examination

Collapsed?

1 **Resuscitate ABCDE** *see p.28–33*

2 **Cervical spine injury?** If injury high on chest wall

Unconscious?

Signs of severe chest injury (seek medical advice)

3
- Difficulty breathing, blue color
- Fast respiratory rate (>30)
- Penetrating wound to chest
- Coughing up blood
- Lack of chest wall movement on one side when breathing
- Severe pain

Treatment

4
- ABCDE assessment (oxygen if available)
- If casualty is shocked, consider tension pneumothorax or hemorrhage—chest decompression may be needed
- Seal any "sucking" hole in chest immediately, with hand if necessary
- Position casualty comfortably and upright
- Insert IV access and consider fluids
- Analgesia, to enable coughing
- Antibiotics if wound is penetrating

Complications

5
- Inability to cough due to pain
- Chest infection
- Blockage of chest drain
- Abdominal injuries due to fractured lower rib (spleen, liver)

Specific chest injuries **6**

Continued monitoring
- Pulse
- Respiratory rate
- Blood pressure
- Temperature
- Urine output
- Chest drain

Watch for Deterioration

Seek medical advice early

1 History and examination

□ ABCDE assessment (*see* p.28–33) takes first priority.
□ Take special care of the neck if there is an injury high on the chest wall.
□ Blue coloration of lips or fingernails is a very bad sign. Seek medical advice immediately.
□ Anticipate problems with breathing, pulse and blood pressure.
□ Get as much information as possible from others about what happened.

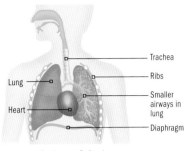

Anatomy of chest

Trachea
Ribs
Lung
Smaller airways in lung
Heart
Diaphragm

Important points in the history

□ How did the accident happen (mechanism of injury)?
□ Shortness of breath
□ Pain in the chest
  – Location?
  – What makes it worse or better?
□ Coughing up blood, sputum?
□ Previous heart or lung disease (asthma/bronchitis)?
□ Other injuries?

Important points in the examination

Look
□ Appearance of casualty (blue/pale)
□ Obvious injuries to chest
□ Look for difference in chest wall movement between each side

Feel
□ Tenderness over chest wall
□ Position of trachea (windpipe)

Listen
□ Harsh or gurgling breath sounds
□ Breath sounds in the chest (with a stethoscope)

Document Breathing rate/vital signs

2 Cervical spine (neck) injury

Injuries high on the chest wall may be associated with injuries to the cervical spine. The bones of the neck may be broken and unstable, but the spinal cord may still be intact. If you are in any doubt at all, immobilize the cervical spine with a semi-rigid collar and a spinal board (*see* pp.178–79).

3 Signs of severe chest injury

□ The casualty may be struggling to breathe and have a high respiratory rate.
□ Low blood pressure may be caused by loss of blood into the chest cavity (hemothorax) or by pressurized air in the chest cavity, compressing the lungs, heart and blood vessels (*see* tension pneumothorax, pp.108–109).
□ Any penetrating wound to the chest is serious and may have damaged lung, heart, blood vessels and even abdominal organs.
□ Coughing up blood indicates damage to both the lung and blood vessels.
□ Lack of movement of one side of the chest in comparison with the other indicates one side does not function properly, probably due to blood or air in the chest cavity. The trachea, which should be in the centerline, may be shifted to the opposite side.
□ Pain is subjective: a stoic casualty may in fact have a serious injury.

④ Immediate treatment

If the casualty is having difficulty breathing or has blue lips or fingers, seek medical advice immediately, and evacuate them as soon as possible. Use oxygen if available.

Chest decompression Possible pneumothorax or hemothorax may call for urgent decompresssion (*see* below and p.194).

Sucking chest wound This type of wound needs to be sealed over immediately, even with a gloved hand, until an appropriate seal can be made (*see* pp.192–93).

Positioning Place the casualty in an upright position. They may need to be wedged in place, particularly in a vehicle. This position is likely to be more comfortable and the lungs function best in an upright position.

IV fluid Fluid may be necessary in cases of significant injury or low blood pressure. Seek medical advice about how much fluid to give.

Analgesia Pain may prevent coughing and deep breathing, so painkillers such as regular acetaminophen, NSAIDs and codeine may be required. Use morphine for severe pain, but seek medical advice first.

Antibiotics If a casualty who has suffered a penetrating open chest wound runs a temperature and starts to cough up green sputum, give antibiotics.

⑤ Complications

Cough If the casualty does not cough often enough, secretions and blood can pool in the lungs, leading to infection and causing breathing difficulties. Encourage the casualty to breath deeply and cough for at least one good stint per hour. Any damaged ribs should be supported during coughing.

Chest infection Treat suspected chest infection (temperature and/or yellow-green sputum) with antibiotics.

Blocked chest drain Chest drains must be monitored very closely as they can easily become blocked, especially if there is blood in the chest. If pressure in the chest rises again, the casualty may collapse. Drains can be flushed with a syringe and sterile saline.

Abdominal injury Fractures to the lower ribs may have also damaged the liver, spleen and other organs.

⑥ Specific chest injuries

Pneumothorax When air collects inside the chest but outside the lungs, this is known as pneumothorax. It may occur spontaneously or may be caused by a blunt injury "bursting" the lung, a fractured rib piercing the lung or a sharp object entering the chest. A small amount of air only makes breathing slightly difficult. If the amount of air increases, it may cause the lungs and heart to "collapse" (a "tension pneumothorax"), necessitating urgent decompression.

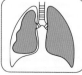

Small pneumothorax
Air collects between lung and chest wall

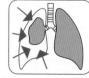

Tension pneumothorax
Trapped air accumulates and compresses lung and heart

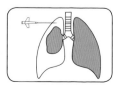

Immediate treatment
Insert cannula and decompress
(*see* **p.194 before doing so**)

Symptoms and signs	Treatment
□ Difficulty in breathing □ Low blood pressure □ The side of the chest not moving (may be difficult to identify) contains the air □ The trachea may be shifted away from the side of the chest with air in it □ Reduced breath sounds on the side of the chest with air in it	□ Without delay, insert a needle or cannula between the ribs in the upper chest on the affected side **(see p.194 before doing so)**. □ A hiss of air may be heard when the needle enters the chest □ Insert a chest drain afterward if available (see pp.195-96)

Hemothorax

Damage to the ribs or blood vessels in the chest may cause bleeding, and the blood may accumulate inside the chest. A significant amount of blood (over 2L) may accumulate, causing the casualty to be shocked and the lung to be compressed.

Symptoms and signs	Treatment
□ Difficulty in breathing □ Casualty may be shocked (low blood pressure) □ Faint breath sounds on affected side	□ If you suspect a hemothorax, seek medical advice □ Insert IV line and give fluid □ Insert chest drain if available

Sucking chest wound

A sucking chest wound may cause deterioration in lung function and there may also be bleeding in to the chest that is not obvious externally.

Symptoms and signs	Treatment
□ Casualty may be distressed, struggling with breathing, have blue lips, low blood pressure □ Obvious hissing/gurgling of air through a chest wound when breathing □ Harsh breath sounds on affected side	□ Cover the hole immediately with a dressing (leaving one side unsealed) or with a gloved hand □ Insert chest drain though hole if possible (see pp.195-96) □ Seek medical advice

Broken ribs and chest wall bruising

Severe bruising and fractured ribs are indistinguishable in the wilderness, but both require rest and adequate pain relief. Broken ribs take up to 6 weeks to heal.

Symptoms and signs	Treatment
□ Tenderness over chest wall at site □ Pain at fracture site if center of chest is pushed in (be gentle) □ The broken ends of bone may be felt grating against each other (crepitus) □ A section of chest wall may move in instead of out when the casualty takes a breath in (a "flail" segment)	□ Analgesia to enable the casualty to breath deeply and cough □ If a flail chest is suspected, give oxygen if possible and seek medical advice □ Do not bind the chest □ Keep comfortable, but mobilize as soon as conditions allow

ABDOMINAL INJURIES

Abdominal injuries such as perforation of the bowel, bruising of the internal organs, and internal hemorrhage (often caused by tearing of the liver or spleen) might be missed if other more obvious injuries distract attention. The kidneys are less likely to be damaged, but are vulnerable to penetrating injuries and significant impact to the flank. Abdominal injuries carry risks of infection and shock. If the situation worsens, the casualty's bowel may stop functioning.

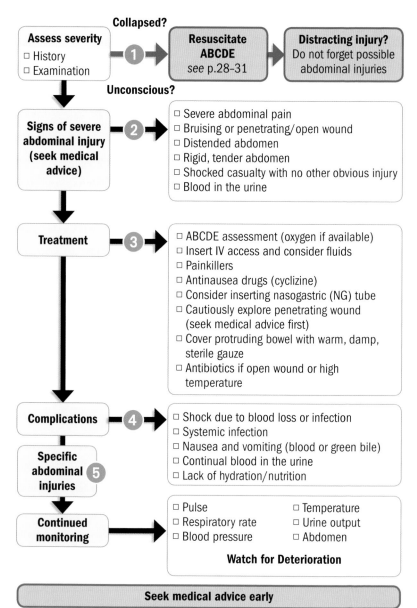

Assess severity
□ History
□ Examination

Collapsed?

❶ **Resuscitate ABCDE** *see p.28–31*

Distracting injury? Do not forget possible abdominal injuries

Unconscious?

Signs of severe abdominal injury (seek medical advice)

❷
□ Severe abdominal pain
□ Bruising or penetrating/open wound
□ Distended abdomen
□ Rigid, tender abdomen
□ Shocked casualty with no other obvious injury
□ Blood in the urine

Treatment

❸
□ ABCDE assessment (oxygen if available)
□ Insert IV access and consider fluids
□ Painkillers
□ Antinausea drugs (cyclizine)
□ Consider inserting nasogastric (NG) tube
□ Cautiously explore penetrating wound (seek medical advice first)
□ Cover protruding bowel with warm, damp, sterile gauze
□ Antibiotics if open wound or high temperature

Complications

❹
□ Shock due to blood loss or infection
□ Systemic infection
□ Nausea and vomiting (blood or green bile)
□ Continual blood in the urine
□ Lack of hydration/nutrition

Specific abdominal injuries ❺

Continued monitoring

□ Pulse   □ Temperature
□ Respiratory rate   □ Urine output
□ Blood pressure   □ Abdomen

Watch for Deterioration

Seek medical advice early

① History and examination

- Internal injuries may not be obvious at first, so reassess often if the casualty is unwell.
- Remember to look at the back of the casualty.
- Penetrating injuries in the chest below the nipples may penetrate the abdomen.
- Lower rib fractures may damage the spleen or liver.

Important points in the history

- How did the accident happen (mechanism of injury)?
- Site and severity of pain?
- Any nausea, vomiting?
- Any blood or bile in vomit?
- Any blood in stool (may be red or tarry black) or urine (may be red or faintly pink)?

Important points in the examination

Look
- Abdominal wounds or bruising (look around the back)
- Abdominal distension
- Old operation scars (appendix, hernia)

Feel
- Any masses in the abdomen
- Tenderness, rigidity

Listen
- Bowel sounds (over lower right side)

Document On abdominal chart

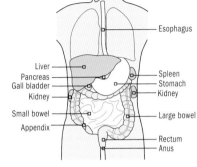

Abdominal organs

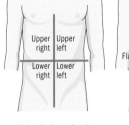

Abdominal quadrants

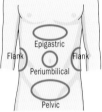

Abdominal regions

② Signs of severe abdominal injury

- The casualty may be sweaty and cold from pain and blood loss.
- A rigid, tense abdomen indicates significant injury.
- Any penetrating wound is serious and may have damaged many internal organs.
- The site and severity of pain gives an indication of which internal organs are damaged (see diagram above) and the possible extent of injury. Note, however, that different people can tolerate different levels of pain and also that the site of pain may be misleading. If the cause of pain is unknown, monitor the casualty closely for signs of deterioration.
- Bruising of the abdomen may not be visible at first. If unsure, re-examine the casualty hourly. Remember to examine the back for penetrating wounds and bruising. Flank bruising may indicate kidney injury.
- The abdomen may look normal at first then become distended over a few hours.
- Bowel sounds (made by gas and liquid being squeezed around) are heard by listening to the abdomen with a stethoscope. If the bowel stops working, there are no bowel sounds, so silence may be a sign of serious injury. Sometimes, however, bowel sounds may be difficult to hear even in a normal abdomen.

③ Immediate treatment

IV fluids Shock should be treated with fluids. Insert an IV cannula (*see* p.186) straight after assessment, to prevent shock worsening, and seek medical advice for guidance on the type of fluids and how much to give.

Analgesia Use acetaminophen, codeine and even morphine for pain. Avoid NSAIDs due to possible complications (bleeding, bowel perforation).

Antinausea medication Vomiting is particularly likely if pain is extreme and if the casualty has been given morphine. The medical kit will contain antinausea drugs. Seek medical advice about which drugs to use and in what order (*see* p.163).

Nasogastric (NG) tube An NG tube may be necessary. Abdominal injury can stop the gut from working properly, causing it to fill up with gastric secretions and become distended, and causing pain to the casualty, who may then vomit. An NG tube attached to a drainage bag (*see* p.200), will allow the stomach contents to pass up the tube into the bag, reducing the risk of distension, pain and vomiting.

Penetrating wounds Wounds of this type are life-threatening: seek medical advice immediately. Explore carefully for foreign bodies, but only after medical advice. Protruding foreign bodies may be plugging a hole in an internal organ or blood vessel, so should not be removed. Clean the wound as far as possible, cover with a sterile dressing, and examine and re-dress every day until evacuation. Report any signs of infection (discharge, bad smell).

Protruding bowel A protruding bowel injury is serious and distressing. Move the casualty to a safe place, cover the bowel with warm, sterile, damp gauze and seek medical advice immediately.

Antibiotics Any penetrating wounds necessitate antibiotics. Administer antibiotics for blunt injuries to the abdomen if the casualty runs a temperature.

④ Complications

Shock If the casualty has lost a significant amount of blood or has a worsening infection, there is a risk of shock. Both of these situations are very serious, and fluid should be administered—preferably by an intravenous route.

Infection Infection may not become evident until a few days after an abdominal injury and may indicate that the bowel is perforated. Use antibiotics for all penetrating injuries and after blunt injuries if the casualty starts to run a temperature or develops signs of peritonitis (*see* p.150).

Nausea and vomiting The casualty may start to vomit hours after the injury or days afterwards. This may indicate deterioration. Use an NG tube to administer antinausea medication. Examine the abdomen for increasing distension, tenderness or any masses. The casualty should not have anything to eat or drink.

Blood in the urine Injury to the kidney or kidneys, the tube from the kidney to the bladder (the ureter), the bladder itself or the tube from the bladder to the outside (the urethra) can all cause blood in the urine. However, in the wilderness, you won't be able to find out precisely where the blood is coming from. The immediate danger is that blood may clot in the bladder, causing retention (a casualty who is unable to pass urine). Seek medical advice before considering passing a catheter, because this may cause complications. Continual blood loss over several days may cause the blood pressure to drop and the casualty may become anemic. Administer fluids and arrange urgent evacuation.

Hydration and nutrition It will be a challenge to maintain hydration and nutrition if a casualty has a distended, painful abdomen and is vomiting; IV fluids may be needed. Fluids can be given via a rectal tube (see p.202), but this is difficult and less fluid will be absorbed. The casualty might need more than 3L of fluid per day after the initial resuscitation—a rate that will exhaust supplies of IV fluid rapidly. Keep in mind that there may be other expeditions in the area with stocks of IV fluids. Monitor urine output for an indication of whether the casualty is adequately hydrated. A urinary catheter may be called for: aim for a urine output of about 0.5-1ml per kilogram of body weight per hour. Seek medical advice for guidance on fluid resuscitation and ongoing fluid requirements.

❺ Sites of pain related to organ injuries

This is a general guide relating the site of injury or maximum pain/tenderness to the internal organs that may be damaged. The site of pain may change over time or become generalized if peritonitis develops, so reassess frequently.

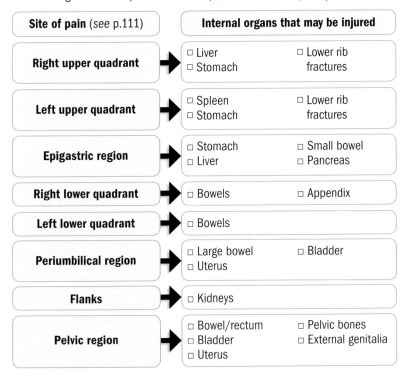

Site of pain (see p.111)	Internal organs that may be injured	
Right upper quadrant	□ Liver □ Stomach	□ Lower rib fractures
Left upper quadrant	□ Spleen □ Stomach	□ Lower rib fractures
Epigastric region	□ Stomach □ Liver	□ Small bowel □ Pancreas
Right lower quadrant	□ Bowels	□ Appendix
Left lower quadrant	□ Bowels	
Periumbilical region	□ Large bowel □ Uterus	□ Bladder
Flanks	□ Kidneys	
Pelvic region	□ Bowel/rectum □ Bladder □ Uterus	□ Pelvic bones □ External genitalia

PELVIC AND HIP INJURIES

Pelvic and hip fractures are usually caused by high energy accidents, such as collisions with vehicles. Injuries to other parts of the body frequently occur at the same time. Falls from heights greater than 2–3m may also injure the spine.

If the pelvis is fractured, the body's organs in the pelvis may be injured as well (bladder, uterus, urethra and blood vessels), causing substantial blood loss. The external genitalia may also be injured, and bleeding from the vagina or penis indicates serious injury. In all cases, seek medical advice at an early stage.

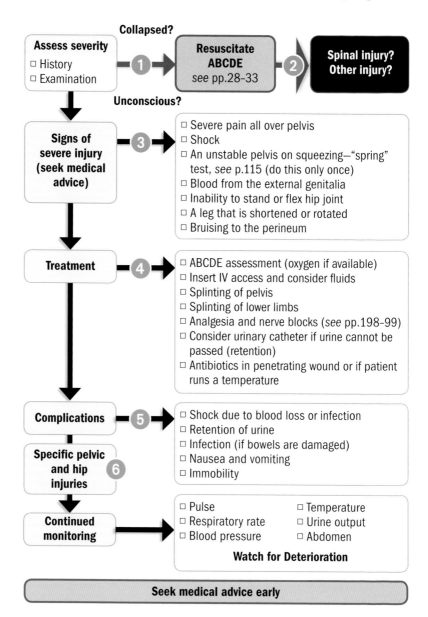

Collapsed?

Assess severity
☐ History
☐ Examination

1 → **Resuscitate ABCDE** see pp.28–33

2 → **Spinal injury? Other injury?**

Unconscious?

Signs of severe injury (seek medical advice)

3 →
☐ Severe pain all over pelvis
☐ Shock
☐ An unstable pelvis on squeezing—"spring" test, see p.115 (do this only once)
☐ Blood from the external genitalia
☐ Inability to stand or flex hip joint
☐ A leg that is shortened or rotated
☐ Bruising to the perineum

Treatment

4 →
☐ ABCDE assessment (oxygen if available)
☐ Insert IV access and consider fluids
☐ Splinting of pelvis
☐ Splinting of lower limbs
☐ Analgesia and nerve blocks (see pp.198–99)
☐ Consider urinary catheter if urine cannot be passed (retention)
☐ Antibiotics in penetrating wound or if patient runs a temperature

Complications

5 →
☐ Shock due to blood loss or infection
☐ Retention of urine
☐ Infection (if bowels are damaged)
☐ Nausea and vomiting
☐ Immobility

Specific pelvic and hip injuries

6

Continued monitoring →
☐ Pulse   ☐ Temperature
☐ Respiratory rate   ☐ Urine output
☐ Blood pressure   ☐ Abdomen

Watch for Deterioration

Seek medical advice early

➊ History and examination

The cause of the accident may indicate the severity of injury. Check for spinal injuries.

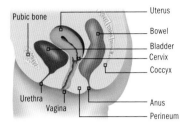

Important points in the history

☐ How did the accident happen?
☐ Site and severity of pain?
☐ Can the casualty stand up?
☐ Any blood in the urine?

Side view of female pelvic organs

Important points in the examination

Look
☐ Obvious deformity of pelvis
☐ Leg shortened or rotated in or out
☐ Bleeding from vagina or penis
☐ Bruising of perineum

Feel
☐ Use the spring test (*see below*) to look for abnormal movement of pelvis
☐ Rigid, tender abdomen

Listen
☐ Bowel sounds in lower right abdomen

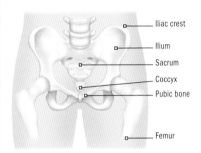

Front view of pelvic area

Pelvic spring test

Pressing down or inward on each iliac crest of a fractured pelvis may cause the pelvis to "open out" or "close in," which may indicate a fracture. Perform this test only once as it may result in further bleeding.

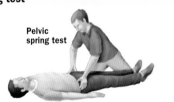

Pelvic spring test

➋ Spinal injury

Falls from heights greater than 2–3m may cause spinal injury. The bones of the spine may be broken, but the spinal cord may still be intact. If in doubt, immobilize the casualty on a spinal board (*see* p.179) and check for other injuries.

➌ Signs of severe pelvic or hip injury

☐ In fractured pelvis, extreme pain. The casualty will be unable to stand.
☐ Rapid blood loss of up to 3L, causing life-threatening shock.
☐ Pelvis fracture may cause damage to the bladder or urethra, indicated by bleeding from the penis or vagina.
☐ Lie the casualty flat and check whether one leg is shorter than the other and rotated inward or outward. Any movement of the hip may be extremely painful and exacerbate bleeding, so do this only once.
☐ Internal bleeding will be indicated by "bruising" to the perineum (the area between the scrotum or vagina and the anus).

4 Immediate treatment

IV fluids Shock should be treated with fluids. Insert an IV cannula (*see* pp.186–87) straight after assessment, to prevent shock worsening, and seek medical advice for guidance on the type of fluids and how much to give.

Analgesia Use acetaminophen, codeine for pain. Avoid NSAIDs initially, which may worsen bleeding. Seek medical advice before using morphine.

Nerve blocks Use local anesthetic injections for pain caused by hip fractures (*see* pp.198–99). They will be effective for a few hours. Repeat as necessary.

Splinting of the pelvis Perform pelvis splinting quickly to reduce blood loss and avoid complications. The procedure is quite simple (*see* illustration below).

Splinting of lower limbs Lower limb splinting is useful for both pelvis and hip fractures (*see* illustration below). Bind the knees and ankles together with padding in-between. Keep the patient flat on their back, with a pillow under their knees.

Urinary catheter If a pelvic fracture damages the urethra or the bladder and prevents the casualty from passing urine, a catheter may be needed. Seek medical advice before inserting a urinary catheter, as there is a risk of further damage.

Antibiotics Infection may not become evident until a few days after the injury and may indicate that the bowel is perforated. Use antibiotics for all penetrating injuries and after blunt injuries if the casualty starts to run a temperature.

5 Complications

Shock If the casualty has lost a significant amount of blood or has a worsening infection, there is a risk of shock. Both of these situations are very serious, and fluid should be administered—preferably by an intravenous route.

Retention of urine Blood clots in the bladder or swelling of damaged tissues may lead to urine retention. Monitor urine output and watch for swelling and pain in the lower abdomen. Suprapubic aspiration may be required (*see* p.202).

Infection May develop gradually and may indicate bowel perforation. Use antibiotics for all penetrating injuries and after a blunt injury if the casualty runs a temperature.

Nausea and vomiting May take hours to develop, indicating injury to the gut. An NG tube should be inserted and antinausea medication given. Look for distension or tenderness in the abdomen. The casualty should take nothing by mouth.

Immobility Initially, the casualty should not move, to reduce the risk of further bleeding, and should be placed in a comfortable, accessible position—wedged in place if in a vehicle. He or she will still need to pass urine (into a bottle) and may need to open the bowels. A bowl and plastic bag might be used as a makeshift bedpan. If the legs and ankles are splinted together, use padding in between.

6 Specific pelvic and hip injuries

Pelvic fracture

Any part of the pelvis may be fractured, and all types of pelvic fracture involve a risk of severe bleeding. Injury to the spine and to other organs in the region may also be present.

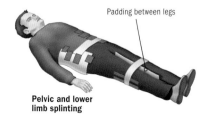

Padding between legs

Pelvic and lower limb splinting

Symptoms and signs	Treatment
□ Severe pain in the pelvic/lower abdominal area □ Unable to stand up or flex hip □ Blood from the vagina or penis □ Bruised perineum □ Positive spring test (see p.115) □ Examine very carefully for other injuries (especially spinal injuries) □ There may be signs of bowel injury (rigid tender abdomen, possibly becoming distended after hours/days)	□ Fluid resuscitation (see pp.184–85) □ Analgesia and antibiotics □ Pelvic splinting □ Lower limb splinting □ Place in an accessible position and wedge in to prevent movement □ Minimize all movement □ Pad all bony prominences and area between splinted legs □ Look for urinary retention; seek advice before inserting a catheter

Hip fracture or dislocation

A hip fracture or dislocation requires a lot of force. Other injuries may also be present. A fractured hip usually causes the leg to rotate outward; a dislocated hip usually causes the leg to rotate inward. The latter is an emergency. The casualty must be evacuated immediately, or an attempt should be made to relocate the dislocation (see p.208). Seek medical advice before doing so.

Symptoms and signs	Treatment
□ Severe pain from the hip or more generalized over the pelvis □ Unable to stand or flex hip □ Inward- or outward-rotated leg □ Possible loss of sensation to leg	□ Fluid resuscitation (see pp.184–85) □ Analgesia □ If dislocation suspected, seek medical advice before relocating □ Lower limb splinting (see opposite)

Urethral injury

The urethra is the tube by which urine passes from the bladder to the outside. It may be damaged by pelvic fracture, preventing urine from being passed.

Symptoms and signs	Treatment
□ Blood from tip of penis or vagina □ Blood in the urine □ Pain passing urine □ Inability to pass urine □ Bruising of the perineum/scrotum □ Full and increasingly painful bladder	□ A urinary catheter might be needed, but seek medical advice □ Suprapubic aspiration might be needed (see p.202) □ Antibiotics if a urethral or bladder injury is suspected

Coccyx injury

Injury to the coccyx can be very painful; it is often impossible to differentiate between bad bruising and a fracture. Fractures may result in long-term pain.

Symptoms and signs	Treatment
□ Pain and tenderness over the base of the spine □ Pain on passing stool	□ Analgesia □ If difficult to pass stool due to pain, use hydration and softening laxatives

LIMBS: FRACTURE AND DISLOCATION

A team member who suffers a fracture may lose a lot of blood and be at risk of shock. Fractures of the femur cause especially heavy bleeding. "Reduce" the fracture (put the ends back together, see pp.206–207) to reduce pain, and apply direct pressure to limit bleeding. When fractures and dislocations threaten the blood and nerve supply beyond the main injury, urgent reduction may be needed (seek medical guidance).

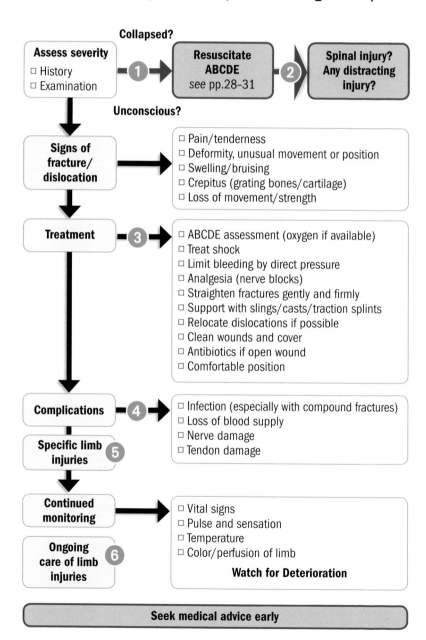

Assess severity
- History
- Examination

Collapsed?

1 → **Resuscitate ABCDE** see pp.28–31

2 → **Spinal injury? Any distracting injury?**

Unconscious?

Signs of fracture/ dislocation
- Pain/tenderness
- Deformity, unusual movement or position
- Swelling/bruising
- Crepitus (grating bones/cartilage)
- Loss of movement/strength

Treatment **3**
- ABCDE assessment (oxygen if available)
- Treat shock
- Limit bleeding by direct pressure
- Analgesia (nerve blocks)
- Straighten fractures gently and firmly
- Support with slings/casts/traction splints
- Relocate dislocations if possible
- Clean wounds and cover
- Antibiotics if open wound
- Comfortable position

Complications **4**
- Infection (especially with compound fractures)
- Loss of blood supply
- Nerve damage
- Tendon damage

Specific limb injuries **5**

Continued monitoring
- Vital signs
- Pulse and sensation
- Temperature
- Color/perfusion of limb

Ongoing care of limb injuries **6**

Watch for Deterioration

Seek medical advice early

1 History and examination

- Femoral fractures may be life-threatening due to blood loss.
- Injuries of the upper limbs are rarely life-threatening.
- However, shoulder and collar bone (clavicle) injuries may be associated with spinal injuries.
- Painful limb injuries may distract from other more serious injuries.

Important points in the history

- How did the accident happen?
- Where and when did it happen?
- Possibility of contamination of wound?
- Any possibility of crushing?
- Any other injuries?
- Any previous fractures or dislocations of the same part?
- Last tetanus injection?

Important points in the examination

Look
- Swelling, bruising
- Deformity
- Open wound over fracture site
- Color of limb

Feel
- Pain, tenderness
- Bone edges
- Crepitus
- Pulses/perfusion beyond fracture
- Sensation beyond fracture

Move
- Ask the casualty to move the limb first, as far as possible in all directions
- Then move the limb yourself very gently, and stop if causing pain

Document findings and vital signs

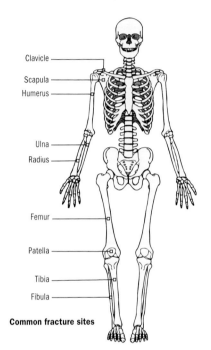

Clavicle
Scapula
Humerus
Ulna
Radius
Femur
Patella
Tibia
Fibula

Common fracture sites

2 Spinal injury

Distracting injuries may divert attention away from spinal damage. Injuries to the shoulder or clavicle (collar bone) may be very painful and can be associated with fractures of the neck. The force required to break the femur may also cause spinal injuries. The bones of the spine may be broken and unstable, but the spinal cord may still be intact. If in any doubt, immobilize the cervical spine (see pp.178–79).

3 Immediate treatment

Limit bleeding Bleeding (external and internal) may cause shock so must be stopped if possible. Apply direct pressure, or attempt to reduce the fracture (see p.206). Use a traction splint to stabilize and reduce a femoral fracture (see p.203), which carries a risk of heavy blood loss.

Analgesia Fractures are very painful, and any attempt at reducing the fracture or dislocation will increase pain, so painkillers are important. Morphine may be required (with antinausea drugs). Nerve blocks may help (see p.199).

Reduce fractures Fractures should be reduced as soon as possible to minimize blood loss and pain. Use firm pressure but do not force (*see* p.206). Muscle spasms might make reduction more difficult, so give analgesia to relax the muscles and sedate the casualty if necessary. Do not attempt reduction more than two or three times as there is a risk of further damage.

Reduce dislocation Shoulders or elbows may need to be relocated to restore blood or nerve supply to the arm, especially if evacuation will take more than a few hours, because the blood or nerve supply to the arm might be cut off. Before and after attempting relocation, check pulses, color, temperature of the arm and sensitivity to touch.

Clean wounds, cover, give antibiotics Treat any wounds near a suspected fracture. The bone may have broken the skin and settled back inside during the accident, causing possible contamination of the bone and tissue; it may still be protruding; or the bone ends may go back under the skin during reduction. Clean thoroughly, cover with a sterile dressing, and start antibiotics immediately.

Splinting/support Splinting or support is needed to reduce pain, bleeding and swelling, whether or not reduction of the fracture or dislocation has succeeded.

Keep in a comfortable position Find a position that does not apply pressure to the dislocation or fracture.

4 Complications

Infection Look for signs of discharge, spreading inflammation, pain or swelling of the skin. If signs of infection are present, seek medical advice on treatment.

Loss of blood supply Blood supply may be cut off immediately or gradually reduced over hours or days. The limb will not survive very long without adequate blood flow—seek medical advice urgently. Treat any signs of shock with appropriate fluid until blood pressure is normal (*see* pp.180–81). Elevating the affected limb may help to reduce swelling, as will rapid reduction of fractures or dislocations. Keep the limb warm.

Nerve damage Damage to nerves may be obvious straight away or become obvious later. Resulting loss of motor function or sensation may be reversible and may improve when the fracture has been reduced. The casualty has the best chances of recovering from nerve damage if fractures or dislocations are rapidly reduced (check nerve function before and after each attempt), shock is treated to restore blood pressure and the limb is raised to reduce swelling.

Tendon damage Damage to tendons cannot be treated in the wilderness. The degree of function loss will depend upon which tendons have been damaged. The casualty may not be able to flex or extend their limb, even using maximum effort. Thoroughly clean any open wounds, treat with antibiotics and splint and immobilize the limb to prevent further injury. Arrange urgent evacuation.

5 Specific upper and lower limb injuries

Types of fracture

In compound ("open") fractures, the bone may be protruding from the wound. It will not be visible in all cases, however—the ends may have gone back under the skin. Treat any fracture with an open wound nearby as compound. In greenstick fractures, the bone bends and then splinters. This type of fracture happens only in children, who have more flexible bones.

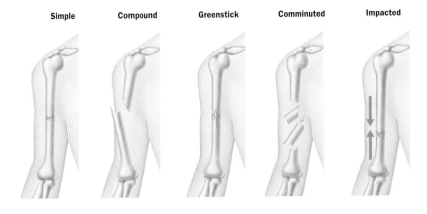

Simple	Compound	Greenstick	Comminuted	Impacted

Clavicle fracture and dislocation

The shaft of the clavicle may fracture or the end that connects to the shoulder may dislocate. These injuries may be caused by a direct blow to the shoulder or by a fall onto the shoulder or an outstretched arm. The bone ends might protrude through the skin.

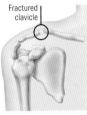

Fractured clavicle

Broken collarbone

Broad arm sling

Symptoms and signs

- Tenderness over clavicle
- Possible deformity (at the outer end over the shoulder if dislocated)
- Tenting of skin over fractured bone ends
- Reduced and painful shoulder movements

Treatment

- Analgesia
- Immobilize and support the arm using a broad arm sling (see above)
- The broken ends of a displaced clavicular fracture may threaten to break the skin. Gentle traction on the arm, pulling away from the center line, may re-oppose the ends, reducing the risk of open fracture.

Shoulder dislocation

Shoulder dislocations are caused by moderate force, such as a fall onto the shoulder or blow to the upper arm. Less force may cause a dislocation if the joint has been dislocated before. The head of the humerus normally dislocates to the front (anteriorly), but may also dislocate downward (the casualty cannot lower their arm) or backward (posteriorly)—the upper arm is rotated toward the midline.

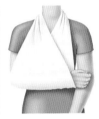

Scapula (shoulder blade)

Socket

Humerus (upper arm bone)

Normal

Artery supplying the arm

Humerus has moved out of socket of joint

Dislocated shoulder

<table>
<tr><td>

Symptoms and signs

- Severe pain
- Restricted movement of arm
- "Squaring" of shoulder (anterior dislocation)
- Loss of blood or nerve supply to arm (pulses and perfusion of skin)
- Crepitus on movement (a sign of possible fracture/dislocation)

</td><td>

Treatment

- Analgesia
- Attempt reduction if blood or nerve supply is reduced (see p.207). Seek medical advice
- Support arm with broad arm sling
- Do not attempt reduction of the fracture if there is crepitus
- Evacuate as soon as possible

</td></tr>
</table>

Humerus, forearm and wrist fractures

These injuries are normally caused by falls onto an outstretched hand or onto the elbow. Blood and nerve supply may be compromised.

<table>
<tr><td>

Symptoms and signs

- Bruising/swelling/deformity
- Loss of movement, crepitus
- Open wounds and bleeding
- Loss of pulses/perfusion/nerve supply to distal limb

</td><td>

Treatment

- Analgesia
- Stop bleeding by direct pressure
- Clean/cover open wounds; antibiotics
- Reduce and splint (see pp.207–208)
- Support with a collar and cuff sling

</td></tr>
</table>

Elbow fracture and dislocation

Dislocation requires considerable force, caused by a direct blow or a fall onto an outstretched hand. It is often combined with a fracture. Blood vessels and nerves to the lower arm all pass close to the elbow joint and may be damaged.

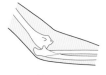

Dislocated elbow

<table>
<tr><td>

Symptoms and signs

- Pain to elbow and lower arm
- Deformity, loss of movement
- Loss of pulses/perfusion/nerve supply to distal limb

</td><td>

Treatment

- Analgesia
- Attempt reduction if blood or nerve supply is reduced (see p.207)
- Support the arm in a broad sling

</td></tr>
</table>

Femoral fracture

Substantial force is required to fracture the femur, such as that generated by falling from a height. Other injuries are common. Seek medical advice immediately.

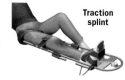

Traction splint

<table>
<tr><td>

Symptoms and signs

- Severe pain
- Shock
- Deformity of the thigh (one side may appear shortened and thicker)
- Loss of movement
- Inability to stand
- Loss of blood and nerve supply to lower leg

</td><td>

Treatment

- Limit external bleeding by direct pressure
- Treat shock with fluids
- Analgesia (consider a femoral nerve block—see p.199)
- Apply traction splint (see p.203)
- Treat open wounds (antibiotics)
- Seek medical advice and evacuate

</td></tr>
</table>

Knee injuries

Knees take a significant pounding on treks and climbs, and occasionally the patella (kneecap) may be become dislocated laterally (away from the midline) or even fractured by a direct blow or sudden flexion. If there is immediate significant swelling and deformity, fracture of the distal femur and dislocation of the knee are possibilities (both require major force). If in any doubt, seek medical advice. For ligament injuries, *see also* pp.126-28.

Symptoms and signs	Treatment
□ Pain □ Swelling around knee □ Inability to perform straight leg raise □ Patella dislocation – Deformity on lateral side of knee – Leg held in slight flexion	□ Analgesia □ Suspected patella fracture – Immobilize with the knee slightly bent, using a full leg splint – Evacuate urgently □ Suspected patella dislocation – Relocate the patella by straightening the leg and pushing the patella back in place firmly with thumbs – Support the knee with crepe or elastic support bandage

Lower leg fractures

Fracture of the tibia is a relatively common injury. A high-energy accident, such as a fall from a height or a vehicle collision, may cause a displaced fracture, in which the bone ends are separated. These are often open. Badly displaced fractures may cause significant swelling of the lower leg, cutting off blood and nerve supply to the distal limb. Urgent evacuation is required.

Symptoms and signs	Treatment
□ Pain at site of fracture □ Deformity □ Swelling (the calf may become very tense over a few hours or days) □ Crepitus □ Loss of distal perfusion and pulses □ Reduced distal sensation □ Inability to bear weight (though it may be possible to weight bear with a fracture of the fibula)	□ Analgesia □ Stop bleeding by direct pressure □ Clean and cover wounds □ Reduce fracture and splint—a traction splint may be effective (*see* p.203) □ Antibiotics for open fracture □ Elevate leg to reduce swelling □ Evacuate urgently if open displaced fracture or significant swelling

6 Ongoing care of fractures and dislocations

□ Keep the casualty comfortable in a position that allows you to examine the wounds easily.
□ Use analgesia to control the pain—more if the casualty is being moved.
□ Elevate the injured limb as much as possible.
□ Watch for limb swelling and check distal perfusion (*see* p.181).
□ Encourage the casualty to mobilize as soon as possible, as pain allows.

HAND, FOOT AND ANKLE INJURIES

The risk of injuries to the hands and feet can be reduced by correct gloves and footwear. Finger dislocations, fractures, crushing and skin loss are among the most common injuries. Deep lacerations may not heal well and often need suturing.

History and examination

Remove rings and bracelets immediately, before swelling occurs. Note that injury to the dominant hand is disabling.

Important points in the history

- How did the accident happen?
- Where and when did it happen?
- Possibility of contamination of wound?
- Any possibility of crushing?
- Other injuries?
- Previous fractures or dislocations of the same part?
- Last tetanus injection?

Important points in the examination

Look
- Swelling; bruising; deformity
- Open wound over fracture site
- Color of toes (with ankle injury)

Feel
- Pain, tenderness
- Bone edges
- Crepitus (bone grating)
- Perfusion beyond fracture
- Sensation beyond fracture

Move
- Check limits of active movement
- Move the hand or foot gently yourself

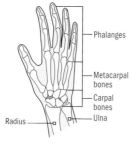

Bones of the hand

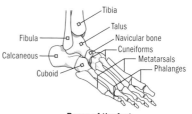

Bones of the foot

Immediate treatment

Stop bleeding Apply direct pressure or put a blood pressure cuff around the forearm or lower leg. After the hand or foot has been inspected, elevated and dressed, remove the pressure cuff immediately to avoid damage caused by lack of blood supply.

Analgesia Consider ring blocks and infiltration for pain relief (see pp.198–99).

Clean wounds, cover and give antibiotics Inspect all wounds for foreign bodies and damage to underlying bones, tendons and nerves.

Reduce or relocate fractures and dislocations See pp.206–209.

Support and elevate Compression bandage, splint, elevation to reduce swelling.

Specific injuries

Hand and foot fractures and crush injuries

Serious hand and foot injuries may require urgent evacuation to prevent loss of vital function. Seek medical advice if there is uncertainty about the severity of the injury.

High arm sling

Symptoms and signs	Specific treatment
□ Deformity, swelling, bruising □ Pain/tenderness/loss of sensation □ Loss of function (strength, movement)	□ Support arm with high arm sling □ Elevate leg and foot □ Splint if necessary

Finger and toe dislocations and fractures

These wounds are often caused by the finger being forced backward or the toe stubbed. Buddy splinting to adjacent finger or toe is usually sufficient immobilization.

Dislocated finger   **Buddy splint**

Symptoms and signs	Specific treatment
□ Deformity □ Swelling, bruising □ Loss of function	□ Reduce dislocation and displaced fracture (see p.208) □ Buddy splint (see above)

Finger and toe crush injuries and de-gloving

Finger and toe injuries are common, especially in the cold, when dexterity and sensation are reduced. Seek medical advice in cases of major tissue loss or amputation.

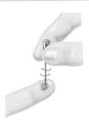

Use a hot, blunt needle to drain a hematoma (see below)

Symptoms and signs	Specific treatment
□ Deformity, bruising and swelling □ Skin loss, exposed bone. In skin loss, look for the missing skin □ Pain, blood under nail (hematoma) □ Possible tissue loss	□ Skin/tissue loss: cover with damp, sterile dressing. Seek medical advice □ Hematoma: heat a blunt needle in a candle flame for 15 seconds. Gently pierce the nail with a rotating motion until blood wells up. Avoid the white base of the nail.

Ankle fracture or dislocation

Fractures of the ankle are relatively common. Dislocations are less common; they are serious and require urgent evacuation.

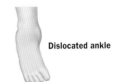

Dislocated ankle

Symptoms and signs	Specific treatment
□ Ankle deformity, worse in dislocation □ Swelling, bruising □ Loss of function □ Severe deformity may cause loss of blood and nerve supply to foot	□ Reduce dislocation urgently if nerve and blood supply are reduced (see p.209) □ Compression dressings and supportive splint (see pp.203–205) □ Elevate leg and foot □ Arrange urgent evacuation

SOFT TISSUE INJURIES

Injuries to muscles, tendons, ligaments, cartilage and bursas go hand in hand with expeditions and physical exertion. Causes include impacts, falls, twists, heavy lifting and repetitive overuse.

Be aware of risks that may contribute to soft tissue injury. Use protective clothing and techniques, and learn how to recognize and treat injuries early.

History and examination

- The injury may be acute (caused by an accident) or chronic (repetitive action)
- Inflammation and infection may complicate injury and need treatment
- The injured part is at risk of further injury
- If in any doubt, treat it as a fracture
- Further investigation may be required

Important points in the history

- When, where, how did it happen?
- Sudden or gradual onset?
- Site and severity of pain?
- Previous similar injuries?

Definitions

Ligament A fibrous rope connecting bones or cartilages, serving to support and strengthen joints
Tendon A fibrous rope attaching the muscle to bone or cartilage
Cartilage A piece of fibrous tissue that forms part of the flexible skeleton
Bursa A fluid-filled lubricating sac situated in places in tissues where friction would otherwise occur.

Important points in the examinations

Look
- Deformity
- Swelling, bruising
- Redness

Feel
- Site of tenderness
- Feel for fluid around joint
- Bone grating if possible fracture
- Warmth of joint (may be infected)

Move
- Ask the casualty to move the injured part, as far as possible, in all directions, testing strength
- Then move the injured part yourself, very gently, stopping if causing pain

Document Findings such as range of movement and what elicits pain

Signs of severe injury

- Severe pain
- Immediate swelling
- Total loss of movement
- Obvious bruising

Immediate treatment

Painkillers NSAIDs reduce pain and inflammation, but use alternative pain relief for the first 24 hours if there is substantial bruising, as NSAIDs may worsen bleeding. Soft tissue injuries will probably not require morphine. Extreme pain usually indicates a more severe injury, such as a fracture.
Rest Rest for 24–72 hours, depending on severity. If this is not possible, immobilize and support the affected joint by taping or splinting (see pp.203–205).
Ice Apply ice to reduce swelling and speed recovery. Avoid direct contact with this skin, as this may cause a cold injury. Apply the pack for 15 minutes 4–6

times a day for 48 hours—longer if having to mobilize with protection/support straight after injury. Alternatives to ice include cold aerosol spray, a cold pack or a cloth soaked in cold water. Combine water and fanning to cool by evaporation.

Compression Use a crepe bandage or elasticated tubular support bandage, especially when mobilizing. This will help to support the injury, reduce further damage and remind the casualty to protect the injured part. Use the correct size to avoid excess compression and reduced blood flow—check blood flow to extremities.

Elevation Raising the limb will also reduce swelling. An injured arm should be held above the heart in a high arm sling (*see* p.205) and an injured leg should be elevated with the foot higher than the hip. Maintain elevation as much as possible.

Mobilization Controlled movement of the injured joint or muscle aids recovery. If mobilizing immediately after injury, protect the injured part with splinting or taping and compression. When mobilizing after 24-72 hours, use a compression dressing, elevate when resting, and resume function gradually.

Specific injuries

Grazes, bruises, rope burns

Symptoms and signs	Treatment
□ Very common, usually very painful □ Potentially contaminated □ Large bruises (hematomas) may become infected and form abscesses	□ Clean thoroughly, remove foreign material, and apply sterile dressing □ Antibiotic cream/ointment/oral □ Abscesses may need incision and drainage (*see* p.197)

Shoulder injuries
Strain may damage the shoulder muscles (rotator cuff). Repetitive actions such as chopping wood, climbing, running and cycling can inflame tendons and bursas.

Symptoms and signs	Treatment
□ Restricted movement □ Pain on movement □ Sudden onset is usually a strain or muscle tear □ Tendonitis/bursitis—gradual onset	□ Rest—immobilization in severe cases (broad arm sling) □ NSAIDs □ Gradual return to activity □ Change method of activity

Elbow and wrist injures
These joints are prone to repetitive strain injury, which causes tenosynovitis. Trauma to the point of the elbow may cause bursitis.

Symptoms and signs	Treatment
□ Restricted movement □ Pain on movement and making a fist □ Swelling over the elbow (bursitis), which feels soft and unstable. Swelling might be tight and painful □ Infection—redness, swelling, warmth	□ Rest and wrist splinting □ Forearm strap for "tennis/golfer's elbow" (not too tight) □ Tight fluid swelling: aspirate with needle/syringe. Seek medical advice □ Antibiotics for signs of infection

Knee injuries

The ligaments, bursas, tendons and cartilage in the knee all serve to stabilize the joint. Any and all can be damaged. Knee injuries may be disabling for weeks and may require evacuation. Repeated kneeling often causes bursitis in front of the knee cap.

Symptoms and signs	Treatment
□ Swelling (the knee may swell rapidly and considerably with severe injury) □ Restricted, painful movement □ Instability on weight bearing is a sign of ligament injury □ "Locking" of the knee on movement is a sign of cartilage damage inside the knee □ Infection—redness, warmth over knee	□ Rest, ice, compression, elevation □ Pain relief (NSAIDs) □ Immobilization (splinting) for serious injury—evacuate □ Aspirate tense swellings with needle and syringe. Seek medical advice first □ Antibiotics for signs of infection □ Careful mobilization as tolerated □ Knee support

Ankle injuries

Injured ankles tend to lose their stability, so take care when mobilizing. It is difficult to tell the difference between a fracture and sprain. In the wilderness, both are treated in the same way. The large Achilles tendon is at the back of the ankle and can be torn or ruptured by a sudden load on the ankle (for example, jumping down from a height). This type of injury is disabling.

Symptoms and signs	Treatment
□ Swelling, bruising □ Pain on movement □ A gap in the Achilles tendon which you may be able to feel □ Cannot stand on tippy toes □ Tenderness over the ankle bones (medial and lateral malleoli)	□ Rest, ice, compression (strapping), elevation □ Pain relief (NSAIDs) □ For suspected Achilles tendon injury, splint ankle and seek medical advice □ Careful mobilization (possible instability)

Lower back pain

Extreme exercise and accidents may injure the back: muscles, ligaments, intervertebral disks and nerves may be involved. Rarely, a back injury may be serious and require evacuation. If in any doubt, seek medical advice.

Symptoms and signs	Treatment
□ What movements make the pain worse or better? □ Where is the pain felt: locally in the back, in the legs, one side or both? □ Previous back problems? **Nerve problems** □ Problems with passing water/feces? □ Burning pain, numbness or tingling felt in the legs?	□ Rest, but encourage early, careful, gentle mobilization □ Care with activities (no heavy lifting, keep back straight) □ Pain relief (NSAIDs) □ Use of low-dose benzodiazepine (diazepam 1–5mg) may help □ If signs of nerve problems, seek medical advice and evacuate

TREATING PAIN

There is no definitive method for assessing pain, so the casualty's own assessment should guide treatment. If a team member tells you they are in pain, believe them.

The adequate provision of pain relief is vital. Pain can be both emotionally debilitating and physically stressful. Limiting pain, on the other hand, promotes physical and emotional recovery, allows proper rest and movement, reduces complications, and speeds healing.

Causes of pain

- Obvious wound
- Fractures
- Infection
- Swelling
- Abscess
- Nerve damage
- Organ infection or damage
- Lack of blood flow to organ (e.g. heart)
- Increased sensitivity (prior nerve damage)

Signs

Usually the casualty will be able to tell you if they are in pain, but confusion, loss of speech or loss of consciousness may prevent this. If the casualty cannot speak, there are signs that indicate the existence and severity of pain.

- Grimacing
- Writhing
- Confusion
- Agitation
- Cold to touch
- Pale
- Sweating
- Nausea, vomiting
- Raised heart rate
- Raised breathing rate
- Deep breathing
- Pain localizing to a point

Treatment

Control acute pain first, then decide on long-term measures for reducing pain to a tolerable level while the casualty heals or until they can be evacuated.

Medications Morphine injected into a muscle provides rapid pain control but may cause nausea, constipation and drowsiness, and should be kept for emergency use. If you do use it, give an antinausea drug at the same time. For longer term pain relief, use regular acetaminophen and NSAIDs (*see* Pain Ladder, inside back cover).

Local anesthesia Give local anesthetic to numb the nerves. This method of pain relief is especially suitable for femoral fractures, finger blocks and repairing wounds (*see* pp.198–199).

Splinting Immobilizes fractures and reduces bone movement, lessening pain.

Reduction Reducing fractures and dislocations will decrease the likelihood of bleeding, swelling and nerve damage.

Elevation Raising an injured limb reduces swelling and pain and allows earlier mobilization.

Cool Sprains and muscle injuries can be cooled to reduce swelling and pain. Burns can also be soothed in this way (*see* p.52).

Warmth/heat Apply heat to minimize muscle pain in the days after an injury. Take care not to cause burns. A hot water bottle wrapped in a towel or a hot compress is ideal.

Dressings Apply dressings to wounds to reduce pain caused by contact.

NEUROLOGICAL DISORDERS

Problems that affect the functioning of the brain can cause headache, behavioral changes, paralysis, loss of consciousness or seizures. Neurological disorders are not always brought on by injury, but may begin without warning.

Epilepsy, migraine and fainting (see p.39) can all occur with no previous sign of abnormality. If the team is at altitude, new onset neurological symptoms may well be caused by high altitude illness (see p.56–61). Symptoms may also be caused by bleeding in and around the brain; infection of the brain or the surrounding membranes (the meninges); blood clots, which may reduce blood supply; low blood pressure; low blood glucose; and lack of oxygen.

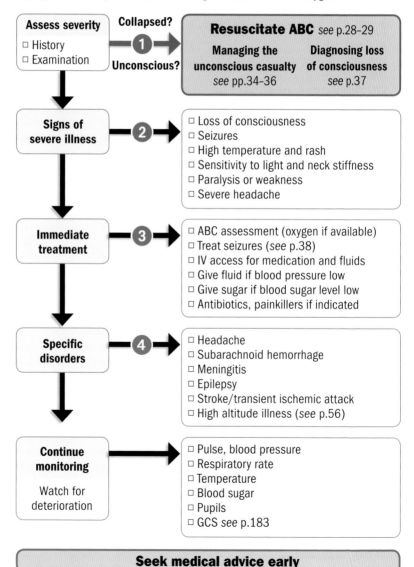

Assess severity
- □ History
- □ Examination

Collapsed?
❶
Unconscious?

Resuscitate ABC see p.28–29

| Managing the unconscious casualty see pp.34–36 | Diagnosing loss of consciousness see p.37 |

Signs of severe illness **❷**
- □ Loss of consciousness
- □ Seizures
- □ High temperature and rash
- □ Sensitivity to light and neck stiffness
- □ Paralysis or weakness
- □ Severe headache

Immediate treatment **❸**
- □ ABC assessment (oxygen if available)
- □ Treat seizures (see p.38)
- □ IV access for medication and fluids
- □ Give fluid if blood pressure low
- □ Give sugar if blood sugar level low
- □ Antibiotics, painkillers if indicated

Specific disorders **❹**
- □ Headache
- □ Subarachnoid hemorrhage
- □ Meningitis
- □ Epilepsy
- □ Stroke/transient ischemic attack
- □ High altitude illness (see p.56)

Continue monitoring

Watch for deterioration
- □ Pulse, blood pressure
- □ Respiratory rate
- □ Temperature
- □ Blood sugar
- □ Pupils
- □ GCS see p.183

Seek medical advice early

① History and examination

- If the casualty is confused, communication may not be possible.
- Use other sources of information: other team members, pre-expedition questionnaires, next-of-kin by mobile or satellite telephone, medic alert bracelets.
- Evaluate regularly—symptoms may develop over time.

Important points in the history	Important points in the examination
- Did the symptoms start suddenly or did they develop over a few days? - Are symptoms related to altitude? - Has this happened before? - Loss of consciousness? - Seizures (generalized/local)? - Severe headache/neck stiffness? - Is speech normal? - Pain when looking at bright light? - Any rashes on the body? - Weakness in arms/legs - Does the casualty take aspirin, clopidogrel, warfarin?	**Look** - Obvious signs of illness—pallor, seizures, rashes anywhere on body? - Pupil size and reaction to light - Oriented in time/place? **Move** - Ask the casualty to move the arms/legs. Is there weakness, paralysis? - Move the limbs gently yourself. Are the limbs unusually stiff or floppy? - Flex head forward gently, touching chin to chest; stop if it hurts

② Signs of severe illness

Loss of consciousness The priority is ABC assessment. See pp.39–41 for causes and treatment.
Seizures Treat seizures that continue for longer than 5 minutes. See p.38 for causes and treatment.
High temperature and rash Temperature and rash indicate infection. The rash does not "blanch" when firmly pressed.
Photophobia Casualty experiences pain looking into a bright light.
Neck stiffness Casualty experiences intense neck pain trying to put chin to chest.
Paralysis or weakness Paralysis may be caused by stroke or hemorrhage. Normally affects one side of the body: legs, arms or one side of the face.
Headache Intense headache may be caused by a subarachnoid hemorrhage, meningitis or a stroke (see below).

③ Immediate treatment (at high altitude—see p.56)

Analgesia Give pain relief for severe headaches: acetaminophen and codeine as required, but not morphine if it can be avoided. NSAIDs may be useful, but not in cases of suspected bleed in the head, as they may worsen bleeding. Use antinausea medication if required—will usually be needed with opiates.
Blood sugar Correct very high or very low blood sugar levels (see p.51).
Antibiotics If there are signs of infection and if there is a possibility of meningitis (see below), use IV route.
Fluids Give extra fluids if the casualty has low blood pressure, but note that fluids may be harmful for certain disorders. Seek medical advice on fluid resuscitation and further hydration.

④ Specific conditions

Headache

Headaches are common and not usually cause for concern. If a headache is severe or lasts longer than 24 hours, despite treatment with plenty of fluids, simple painkillers and rest, treat as serious.

CAUSES OF HEADACHE

Meningitis	→ See opposite page
Subarachnoid hemorrhage	→ See opposite page
Carbon monoxide poisoning	→ See p.170

LESS SERIOUS, MORE COMMON CAUSES

Symptoms and signs	Treatment
Tension/Tiredness □ General headache and sore neck □ Lack of sleep □ Dehydration	□ Efficient rest □ Good hydration □ Change of tasks or routine □ Analgesia
Dehydration □ Thirst □ Lethargy, fatigue □ Small amount of dark urine □ Heavy work, sweating □ Tropical climate/cold, dry climate	□ Attention to drinking plenty of rehydration fluids, especially in hot climates and when working hard □ Work as a team to keep hydrated □ Watch color of urine—if it goes dark, drink more rehydration fluid
Sinusitis □ Tender over cheek or eyebrow □ Fever □ Foul discharge from nose or back of throat	□ Antibiotics □ Analgesia □ Avoid blowing nose □ Steam inhalation may help □ No diving or air travel
Migraine □ Previous history of migraine? □ Pain is usually on one side of head □ Visual disturbances (blurring, flashing lights, even blindness)	□ Analgesia □ Rest in quiet and dark □ Keep hydrated □ Antinausea medication if sick □ Avoid chocolate, citrus fruits, cheese
Sunstroke □ History of sun exposure without proper protection □ Heavy work in direct sun □ Reddened, painful, itchy skin, blistering	□ Keep out of sun □ Wear sunscreen, hat, shirt □ Cool down (damp clothes, hat) □ Analgesia □ Keep hydrated □ Antinausea medication if sick
Alcohol/drugs □ History of heavy alcohol intake □ Nitrates (nitroglycerin spray) □ Dehydration	□ Avoid certain prescription drugs if they are possibly the cause—seek medical advice □ Moderate alcohol intake

Subarachnoid hemorrhage (SAH)

A SAH occurs when a blood vessel ruptures in the head. This is a life-threatening event and may cause sudden loss of consciousness and death.

Symptoms and signs	Treatment
□ Sudden onset severe headache —like a blow to the back of head □ Confusion, drowsiness □ Neck pain, vomiting □ Seizures/loss of consciousness	□ Assess ABC (see p.28–29), oxygen □ Treat seizures (see p.38) □ Analgesia and rest □ Seek medical advice □ Urgent evacuation

Meningitis

Inflammation of the membrane covering the brain is known as meningitis. Usually caused by infection, this condition is life-threatening if it is not recognized quickly and treated with antibiotics. Consider immunization of team members before departure.

Symptoms and signs	Treatment
□ Fever and headache for several hours □ Stiff neck □ Photophobia □ Possibly a nonblanching rash □ Later—unconsciousness, shock	□ Assess ABC (see p.28–29), oxygen □ Antibiotics (preferably IV) □ Analgesia for headache, sore neck □ Seek medical advice □ Urgent evacuation

Epilepsy (for control of seizures—see p.38)

Known epilepsy sufferers may be carrying medication, but if they suffer any sickness, oral medication may not be absorbed and seizures may result. After the seizure, the casualty will be drowsy (the "post-ictal" period—see p.38).

Symptoms and signs	Treatment

□ Generalized or localized seizures
□ Incontinence, tongue biting
□ Causes:
  - Non-absorption of normal meds
  - Infection
  - Alcohol withdrawal
	□ Assess ABC (see p.28–29), oxygen
	□ Prevent injury but do not restrain
	□ Recovery position
	□ Treat seizures (see p.38)
	□ Seek medical advice
	□ Urgent evacuation

Stroke and transient ischemic attack (TIA)

Strokes and TIAs are caused by blood clots in the brain. Both disorders manifest in a similar way, but the symptoms of TIA should resolve in an hour or so. Both events can threaten life.

Symptoms and signs	Treatment
□ Paralysis down one side of the body, one limb or side of face □ Difficulty speaking and swallowing □ Visual problems □ Altered sensation/poor coordination □ Headache and possible seizures	□ Assess ABC (see p.28–29), oxygen □ Treat seizures (see p.38) □ Recovery position if unconscious □ Analgesia if required □ Seek medical advice □ Urgent evacuation

EYE DISORDERS

Serious eye problems are quite rare, as the eye socket and eyelid afford a good degree of protection. However, extreme environments can irritate eyes: wind, snow, UV glare, fatigue and lack of hygiene all pose risks, particularly for wearers of contact lenses or glasses. See pp.102–105 for eye trauma.

There are only limited options for treating eye disorders in the wilderness, but antibiotic drops or ointment, anesthetic drops, eye lubrication, rest and protection will successfully treat most complaints. If a team member has become blind or has a painful red eye, seek immediate medical advice and arrange evacuation.

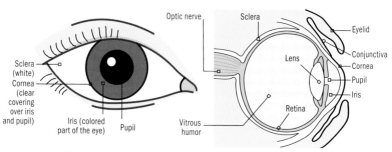

Front view of the eye

Side view of the eye

Signs of severe illness

- ☐ The team member may have a history of eye problems, which should give you some idea of the diagnosis.
- ☐ Examination needs to be done in a safe and stable place, and the area should be well lit (for example, with a headlamp).
- ☐ Compare eyes to see if the problem affects both sides.

Important points in the history

- ☐ How quickly have the symptoms developed?
- ☐ Pain? Worse with light?
- ☐ Blurred, poor, or double vision?
- ☐ Any discharge from eye (stickiness)?
- ☐ Previous problems with eyes/vision?
- ☐ Eye surgery in past (cataract/laser)?
- ☐ Contact lenses or glasses?
- ☐ Diabetes, glaucoma, arthritis?
- ☐ Medications for eyes?

Important points in the examination

Look (compare sides)
- ☐ Redness over sclera, discharge?
- ☐ Swellings around eye and lids?
- ☐ Size and reactivity of pupil?
- ☐ Blood or pus in front of the iris?
- ☐ Cloudiness of cornea or lens (pupil should appear clear black)
- ☐ Inside eyelids? (see pp.102-103)

Feel (compare sides)
- ☐ Press gently on globe of eye —painful or very tense?
- ☐ Tenderness around orbit, eyelids?

Move
- ☐ Ask casualty to look at your finger held 30cm away. Move finger up/down and side to side slowly. Keep head still. Ask about double vision and watch eye movements closely.
- ☐ Record which movements cause pain

Visual acuity
- ☐ Test vision by reading small text from a book at normal distance

Using fluorescein drops to help examination of the eye

Fluorescein dye will stain any abrasion or ulceration of the cornea a greenish color when lit by bright, preferably blue, light.

□ Put a few drops of tetracaine 0.5% local anesthetic inside the lower eyelid (fluorescein dye will sting).

□ After two minutes, put in a few drops of fluorescein inside the lower eyelid.

□ Close the eye for a minute or so and wipe off excess fluorescein.

□ Examine the cornea with a magnifying glass and bright light (blue if available).

□ To minimize complications caused by an adverse reaction, stain the eyes one at a time, 30 minutes apart.

Signs of severe eye disorders

Blindness: In one eye or both; may or may not be painful
Reduction in visual acuity: Blurred vision
Red eye: Particularly when the eye is painful (see below)
Unreactive pupil: When a bright light is shone into the eye
Cloudy cornea or lens: The pupil should be clear black

▶ **Seek medical advice**

Causes of "red eye"

Serious
□ Acute glaucoma—blurred vision, painful eye
□ Acute iritis—blurred vision, pain, photophobia
□ Corneal inflammation/ulceration (keratitis)
□ Orbital cellulitis—swelling and redness around the eye
□ Trauma to the eye (see pp.104–105)

▶ **Seek medical advice**

Less serious
□ Prolonged contact lens use
□ Conjunctivitis/scleritis
□ Snow/sea blindness
□ Subconjunctival hemorrhage
□ Foreign body in the eye (see p.104)

Specific conditions

Contact lens problems

Caring for contact lenses in the wilderness is not easy. They are more difficult to clean, more difficult to replace and may be damaged by exposure to sun, wind, sand, sea and salt. Take extras or use daily disposables.

□ Lens stuck in eye: wash out with copious sterile saline; someone may need to help by extracting the lens gently.

□ Sore, dry eyes: See p.136.

□ Conjunctivitis: stop wearing the lenses until infection completely clears; sterilize lenses and use antibiotic eye drops.

□ Corneal abrasion: a problem with prolonged use. Stop wearing lenses; for treatment, see p.104.

□ Lost lens: may still be in the eye but difficult to see. Inspect the inside of the lids thoroughly, particularly the upper lid (see p.103).

Dry eyes

Dry eyes result from exposure to sun, wind and dry environments. Contact wearers are particularly at risk.

Symptoms and signs	Treatment
□ Eyes are red, painful and feel gritty □ Both eyes usually affected □ Long period of wearing contact lens	□ Artificial tears (e.g. hypromellose) □ Reduce time wearing contact lenses □ Sunglasses/goggles to protect eyes □ Antibiotic ointment may lubricate the eyes and help to relieve pain

Snow/sea blindness (ultraviolet keratitis)

This disorder is caused by UV rays and is a marked risk on snow and water due to reflection. The "blindness" is caused by eye spasm, watering and eyelid swelling.

Symptoms and signs	Treatment
□ May happen after only 2–3 hours of exposure □ Very painful gritty, red eyes □ Face may be burnt red as well □ Bright light may hurt eye □ Headache is common □ Usually both eyes affected □ Eyelids may be swollen	□ Sunglasses with side protection □ Assess for foreign bodies first □ Local anesthetic drops for pain, and oral painkillers for headache □ Antibiotic ointment may lubricate the eyes and help to relieve pain □ Use eye patch for 24 hours then reassess (earlier if discharging)

Conjunctivitis

Conjunctivitis is a serious problem because other team members may catch it. Do not share towels or bedding. One eye may be affected, but usually both are.

Symptoms and signs	Treatment
□ Red, painful eye (cornea is not red) □ Discharge of pus—bacterial infection □ Watery discharge—viral infection □ Itchy eye—allergic cause □ Vision not affected	□ Antibiotic drops or ointment for 5 days □ Viral conjunctivitis will clear without treatment □ Antihistamine eye drops if allergic cause suspected

Corneal inflammation/ulceration (keratitis)

Keratitis may cause scarring, which can permanently affect vision. Causes include infection, contact lens overuse and corneal abrasion. Do not use steroid drops if there is any possibility of corneal infection—this may worsen inflammation.

Symptoms and signs	Treatment
□ Red and painful eye □ Photophobia □ Watering □ Cloudy cornea with bacterial infection □ Blurred vision	□ Ulcers will glow greenish with fluorescein staining □ Antibiotic drops or ointment □ Seek medical advice as vision may be threatened

Subconjunctival hemorrhage

Symptoms and signs	Treatment
□ One eye may appear alarmingly red □ Vision unaffected □ No apparent cause (minor trauma, use of drugs such as aspirin, warfarin)	□ No specific treatment required □ Should clear in 2–3 weeks □ If recurrent, check blood pressure and review medications

Orbital cellulitis

Inflammation of the orbit within which the eye sits is a threat to eyesight. Administer antibiotics by an IV route.

Symptoms and signs	Treatment
□ Painful, red eye □ Swelling around eye, possibly causing lids to close □ Possible loss of vision □ Fever and feeling unwell	□ IV antibiotics □ Hydration □ Analgesia as required □ Seek medical advice immediately □ Arrange urgent evacuation

Acute glaucoma

A buildup of fluid pressure within the eye may threaten sight. Usually, only one eye is affected. Pilocarpine 0.5% drops may be available for emergency treatment.

Symptoms and signs	Treatment
□ Pain, nausea, vomiting □ Red eye around the cornea, which might be hazy □ Blurred vision, halos □ Semidilated/unresponsive pupil □ History of glaucoma/other problems	□ Pilocarpine 0.5% eye drops in affected eye every 15–30 minutes—pupil will constrict □ Rest and sit upright □ Antinausea drugs if needed □ Seek medical advice and evacuate

Acute iritis (acute uveitis)

The casualty may have a history of iritis and may have a disease such as arthritis.

Symptoms and signs	Treatment
□ Sudden onset of pain □ Reddened eye around cornea □ Watering eyes, blurred vision □ Photophobia □ Small, possibly irregular pupil	□ No specific treatment in wilderness □ Rest, analgesia □ Steroid eye drops may help, but seek medical advice □ Urgent evacuation

Eyelid infections

Symptoms and signs	Treatment
□ Stye: small boil arising from eyelash follicle—may discharge naturally □ Chalazion: infected gland in eyelid, which may develop into an abscess or nodule affecting vision	□ "Hot spooning": wrap warm, damp cloth around small spoon and press to eye; repeat every few hours □ Antibiotic ointment or drops □ Chalazion may need surgery

DENTAL AND MOUTH DISORDERS

A dental problem or mouth ulcer can incapacitate the person who has developed the problem. All team members should have a dental checkup some weeks before departure, particularly if the expedition is to a remote area.

The medical kit should contain a standard dental repair set, which will include such items as temporary filling material and basic dental tools. Control of symptoms such as pain, swelling and infection is the other element of treatment. Only extract teeth if it becomes absolutely necessary.

History and examination

- □ Examination needs to be done in a safe and stable place that is well lit (with a headlamp, for example).
- □ Procedures are easier if they are carried out from behind the head.
- □ Sinusitis may resemble dental pain. Conversely, dental pain is sometimes felt in the face and ears.

Important points in the history

- □ Site and severity of pain?
- □ Fever, feeling unwell?
- □ History of trauma?
- □ Any foul tasting discharge or smell from mouth or nose?
- □ Retrieve knocked out teeth/ dentures
- □ Previous dental problems?

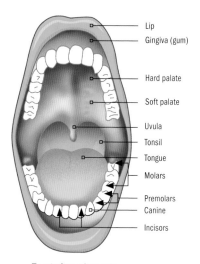

Lip
Gingiva (gum)
Hard palate
Soft palate
Uvula
Tonsil
Tongue
Molars
Premolars
Canine
Incisors

Front view of mouth

Important points in the examination

Look
- □ Inspect all teeth—note crowns/ fillings
- □ Check gums, tongue (above and below) and lips for inflammation, swelling and discharge

Feel
- □ Check each tooth for looseness, tenderness
- □ Examine lips, tongue, cheeks for tenderness, swelling, ulcers
- □ Tap the area over the cheek below the eye and the forehead above it, checking for sinusitis

Document findings for each tooth

Replacing a filling

- □ Stable working position; good light; use cotton wool swabs to keep tooth/ hole dry
- □ Gently probe cavity, remove loose filling bits
- □ Push in small amount of filling mix from dental kit (for mixing, follow instructions)
- □ Pack in firmly and repeat to fill hole (do not leave raised above tooth surface)
- □ Bite together with damp cotton wool pad between teeth for a few minutes

Specific conditions

Toothache

Symptoms and signs	Treatment
□ May result from cracked tooth or dislodged filling □ Pain on drinking cold/hot drinks □ Pain in tooth or cheek; earache □ May result in root or gum abscess	□ Analgesia □ Antiseptic mouthwash □ Antibiotics in fever and local inflammation □ Replace filling if lost (see p.138)

Root and gum abscesses

Symptoms and signs	Treatment
□ Pain/swelling/inflammation of gum □ May discharge into mouth □ May spread to cause swelling of cheek, difficulty in opening mouth —this is an emergency	□ Oral antibiotics, analgesia □ Antiseptic mouthwash □ Lancing the abscess may be possible if it is tense or pointed □ Seek medical advice if it worsens

Broken or knocked out (avulsed) teeth

Symptoms and signs	Treatment
□ Try to find tooth and keep it in saliva/milk; aim to re-implant within 30 minutes □ Do not handle root of tooth □ Check for other injuries □ Splint broken tooth as for avulsed tooth	□ Clean tooth/socket with sterile saline □ Reimplant to same height as other teeth—hold in place for 10 minutes □ Splint with tin foil wrapped over teeth or filling material squeezed in-between thoroughly dried teeth □ Analgesia and antibiotics

Broken crowns, bridges and dentures

Symptoms and signs	Treatment
□ There are different types of crowns □ Bridges are also varied and are usually impossible to replace □ Denture wearers should take a spare set; a superglue repair may not be successful	□ It may be possible to reglue a crown—get dental advice □ Clean and dry both surfaces, and use dental glue from the kit □ Sensitive sockets may require temporary filling for protection

Mouth ulcers and cold sores

Symptoms and signs	Treatment
□ May result from trauma (teeth) □ Bacterial infection: bleeding gums and bad breath □ Herpes infection: lots of small ulcers	□ Bacterial infection: antibiotics, antiseptic mouthwash □ Cold sores/Herpes virus: oral acyclovir cream early

EAR, NOSE AND THROAT DISORDERS

Infections of the ears, nose and throat (ENT) are particularly prevalent if conditions are cold, tiring and damp. The goal of treatment is to relieve symptoms. The infection is usually viral, in which case it will clear without action. For bacterial infection (indicated by a discharge of pus), administer antibiotics.

Foreign bodies can enter the various tubes and spaces in the head and lodge there. This can cause complications. Diving, air travel and rapid ascent to altitude may cause pain or rupture of the eardrum (barotrauma) and pain in the sinuses, if they are blocked. A bleeding nose may seem insignificant, but can become life-threatening if loss of blood continues unchecked.

History and examination

☐ Examination needs to be performed in a safe and stable place with good light (from a headlamp, for example).
☐ Compare sides.
☐ Do not stick things into the ear, apart from an otoscope. If you do use one, you should make sure you know how to use it the correct way.

Important points in the history

☐ Site and severity of pain?
☐ Is pain worse if you: try to exhale with nose blocked/mouth closed; blow nose; tap cheek/forehead?
☐ Feeling of deafness?
☐ Feeling of object stuck in throat?
☐ History of ENT problems?

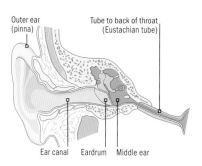

Front view of ear

Important points in the examination

Look (compare sides)
☐ In ears, up nose, in mouth using good light (otoscope to examine ears if available)
☐ Pus in ears, on tonsils, in nose
☐ Inflamed tonsils, throat, ear canal
☐ Foreign bodies, wax in ears
Feel
☐ Tap on cheek and forehead—painful with sinusitis

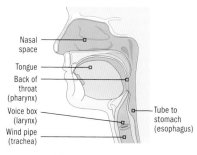

Side view of nose and mouth

Using an otoscope

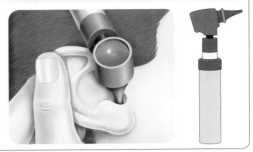

- □ Use an otoscope carefully—stop if you are causing pain
- □ Gently pull the outer ear upward and back, to straighten out the canal
- □ Use a clean tip for each ear and each patient

Specific conditions

Buildup of earwax

Symptoms and signs	Treatment
□ Gradual onset of deafness	□ A few drops of olive oil (or ear drops) each day for a few days □ Do NOT use cotton swabs □ May need aspirating by doctor

Outer ear infection

Symptoms and signs	Treatment
□ Pain and discharge from ear □ Inflamed ear canal, possibly blocked with wax, secretions, swelling □ Pulling on the outer ear hurts □ Feels unwell if severe infection	□ Antibiotic ear drops □ If severe—oral antibiotics □ Gentle cleaning of ear with sterile water □ Avoid diving, swimming, air travel

Middle ear infection

Symptoms and signs	Treatment
□ Pain and deafness □ May feel unwell with cough, cold □ Inflamed eardrum visible through otoscope □ Eardrum may "pop"—relief of pain, purulent discharge	□ Oral antibiotics □ Painkillers □ Decongestant (pseudoephedrine) may be helpful □ Avoid diving, swimming, air travel

Ear barotrauma

Symptoms and signs	Treatment
□ Pain in ear with changing pressure when Eustachian tube blocked □ Eardrum may be red and inflamed □ Drum may rupture—blood from ear □ If dizzy and sick, seek medical advice	□ Painkillers □ Oral antibiotics if ruptured drum □ Avoid diving, swimming, air travel until better

Foreign bodies in ear, nose and throat (may need medical help)

Symptoms and signs	Treatment
Ear Deafness, discharge, irritation; an insect may cause buzzing in ear **Nose** Discharge, irritation; danger of inhalation of foreign body **Throat** Coughing, wheezing, may cause choking (see pp.42-43); object often stuck at back of tongue, in tonsils; feeling of object in throat may persist	**Ear** Olive oil may soften the object; attempt to remove under direct vision; do not persist and cause injury to canal **Nose** Try to blow out first or remove under direct vision—may need help if far back in nose **Throat** Use tongue depressor and direct vision—use forceps

Sinusitis

Symptoms and signs	Treatment
□ Pain on tapping over cheek below eye, or over forehead above eyebrow □ Fever, headache □ Purulent discharge into nose/throat	□ Oral antibiotics □ Painkillers □ Nasal decongestants

Sore throat and tonsillitis

Symptoms and signs	Treatment
□ Fever, headache □ Some difficulty swallowing □ Tonsillitis—inflamed tonsils, at either side of mouth at back of tongue (use tongue depressor), sometimes with pus visible	□ Use acetaminophen, ibuprofen □ Tonsillitis may require antibiotics □ Do not use amoxicillin (or amoxicillin + clavulanate) —may cause rash □ If cannot swallow fluids, seek medical advice if dehydrated

Nose bleeds

Symptoms and signs	Treatment
□ May be common at altitude □ Shock may develop with continual bleeding □ Most bleeds are from inside the front part of the nose □ Bleeds from the back of nose are more serious (difficult to control) □ Blood may be swallowed, so not seen on outside □ Check for medications such as warfarin, aspirin, clopidogrel—if the casualty is on these, seek medical advice	□ Sit up; do not swallow blood □ Firmly squeeze soft part of nose for 10 minutes; reassess; reapply pressure if needed □ In continued bleeding, cut a ribbon of gauze, soak in paraffin ointment/petroleum jelly; pack firmly into nose, but leave a tail for removal; remove at 48 hours; seek medical help □ In catastrophic bleeding, pass a lubricated urinary bladder catheter to back of nose, inflate balloon, and pull firmly forward—only with medical advice

CHEST DISORDERS

People of all ages now take part in expeditions. Older team members are more susceptible to heart and lung problems, particularly in situations of intense physical exertion and at high altitude. Even team members who seem to be in good shape might develop unforeseen problems in arduous conditions.

The onset of symptoms at altitude may well be due to high altitude illness—see p.56. Even the fittest members of the expedition can be at risk from this.

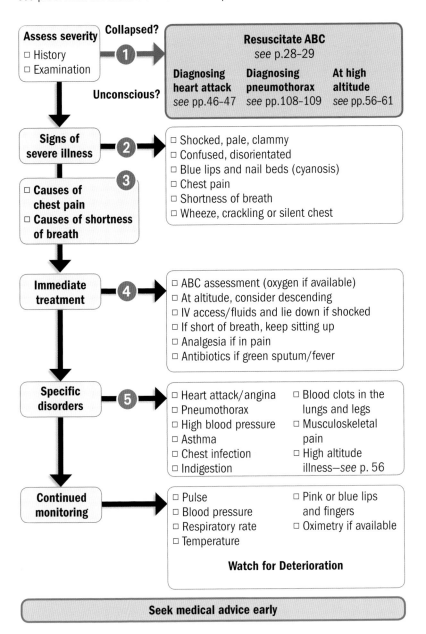

Assess severity
☐ History
☐ Examination

Collapsed? ➊

Unconscious?

Resuscitate ABC
see p.28-29

Diagnosing heart attack	Diagnosing pneumothorax	At high altitude
see pp.46-47	see pp.108-109	see pp.56-61

Signs of severe illness ➋

Causes of chest pain
☐ **Causes of shortness of breath** ➌

☐ Shocked, pale, clammy
☐ Confused, disorientated
☐ Blue lips and nail beds (cyanosis)
☐ Chest pain
☐ Shortness of breath
☐ Wheeze, crackling or silent chest

Immediate treatment ➍

☐ ABC assessment (oxygen if available)
☐ At altitude, consider descending
☐ IV access/fluids and lie down if shocked
☐ If short of breath, keep sitting up
☐ Analgesia if in pain
☐ Antibiotics if green sputum/fever

Specific disorders ➎

☐ Heart attack/angina
☐ Pneumothorax
☐ High blood pressure
☐ Asthma
☐ Chest infection
☐ Indigestion
☐ Blood clots in the lungs and legs
☐ Musculoskeletal pain
☐ High altitude illness—see p. 56

Continued monitoring

☐ Pulse
☐ Blood pressure
☐ Respiratory rate
☐ Temperature
☐ Pink or blue lips and fingers
☐ Oximetry if available

Watch for Deterioration

Seek medical advice early

1 History and examination

□ ABC assessment takes priority over everything (*see* p.28-29).
□ A blue or very pale casualty is a very bad sign—seek medical advice immediately.
□ The casualty may have a history of heart or lung problems.
□ Determine what medications the casualty is taking.

Important points in the history	Important points in the examination
□ Did the symptoms start suddenly or develop over a few days? Were they associated with ascent to altitude? □ Pain in the chest: - Location (up to jaw, down arms?) - Severity (worst ever?) - What makes it better or worse? □ Shortness of breath: - Did anything make it worse? - Did anything obvious bring it on? - Able to speak in sentences or just one or two words? □ Sputum (amount and color) □ Pain/swelling of legs □ Recent immobility/air travel □ Any history of similar attacks □ Usual medications	**Look** □ Appearance of casualty (blue/pale/feverish/sweaty) □ Obviously struggling with breathing, perhaps sitting upright leaning forward □ Tender swelling of calves **Feel** □ Pulse, perfusion □ Tenderness over chest wall □ Position of trachea (windpipe) **Listen** □ Breath sounds in the chest using a stethoscope (present or absent?) □ Harsh or crackly breath sounds **Document** Vital signs, peripheral perfusion

2 Signs of severe illness

Pale and clammy skin Extreme pain or low blood pressure can affect the skin in this way. Conditions that cause these symptoms include include heart attack (*see* pp.46-47), pneumothorax (*see* pp.108-109) and severe indigestion (*see* p.151).

Confusion, disorientation
If thoughts are muddled, possible causes include low blood pressure, shortage of oxygen and infections, such as meningitis, (*see* p.133).

Blue lips or nails If the casualty's circulation is adversely affected by lack of oxygen or low blood pressure, the lips or nails may turn blue.

Chest pain Pain may be felt in various locations in the chest. Heart problems usually cause crushing pain in the center of the chest, in the jaw and/or down the left arm.

Anatomy of chest

Shortness of breath Breathing may be faster and/or deeper. If breathing problems are severe, the casualty will be sitting up, leaning forward, bracing themselves with their arms and obviously laboring.

Wheezing Asthma is the most common cause of wheezing. Heart problems and chest infections can also cause whistling, rattling breath.

Crackling Crackling sounds are another breathing abnormality associated with chest infection or heart problems.

Silent chest The absence of chest sounds through a stethoscope is grave in a casualty who is having difficulty breathing. Seek medical advice immediately.

❸ Causes

Causes of shortness of breath	
□ Asthma	□ Pulmonary embolus (clot in lungs)
□ Anxiety	
□ Pneumothorax	
□ Heart problems	□ Chest infection
□ Trauma	□ High altitude

Causes of chest pain	
□ Heart attack	□ Chest infection
□ Indigestion	□ Pulmonary embolus
□ Angina	
□ Anxiety	□ Trauma
□ Pneumothorax	□ High altitude

❹ Immediate treatment (high altitude—*see p.56*)

If breathing is labored and the casualty's circulation is compromised (indicated by blue lips or fingers), seek medical advice immediately, and start to arrange for immediate evacuation/descent if possible. Use oxygen if available.

Shock Treat shock immediately. Lie the casualty down and prop the legs up above the heart. Insert an IV cannula and give fluids—500ml initially, then check blood pressure (*see* illustration, right, and pp.186-87). Seek medical advice immediately.

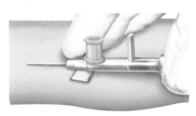

Inserting an IV cannula

Shortness of breath Keep the casualty sitting up—the lungs work better in this position. Administer oxygen if available. Investigate the cause of breathlessness—see list above and signs/symptoms and treatments of specific conditions.

Chest pain Treat chest pain: morphine IM injection if pain is extreme (*see* illustration, right, and p.189), otherwise acetaminophen and NSAIDs (check the casualty has no stomach ulcer or asthma problems first). Investigate the

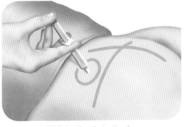

IM injection in buttock

cause—*see* list above and signs/symptoms and treatments of specific conditions.

Antibiotics Use antibiotics if there is fever and green sputum—IV if the casualty looks unwell, has a temperature above 102°F (39°C) and is short of breath.

⑤ Specific conditions

Pneumothorax	➜	See pp.108-109
Indigestion	➜	See pp.151
High altitude illness	➜	See pp.56-61

Heart attack/angina

Team members who smoke, who have high blood pressure or diabetes or who have had previous angina or heart attacks are all at increased risk. Risk also increases with age. Angina is the early stage of heart disease. It is usually triggered by physical exertion and should stop when the casualty rests. Any team members who suffer from angina should be seen, fully assessed and treated by a doctor before departure. They may be unwise to take part in expeditions to cold climates and isolated areas.

Symptoms and signs	Treatment
☐ Central, crushing chest pain—may also be felt in the left or right arm, jaw, neck and abdomen ☐ Heart attack pain is continuous ☐ Angina pain improves with rest ☐ Sweating, pale, short of breath ☐ Nausea and vomiting ☐ Possible collapse from either low or very high blood pressure	☐ If any doubt, treat as a heart attack (see pp.46-47) ☐ Give oxygen if available ☐ Treat pain with morphine 5-10mg IM injection if very severe, sweaty ☐ Nitroglycerin spray under tongue ☐ If in any doubt, give aspirin 300mg ☐ Rest and avoid exertion and stress ☐ Seek medical advice and evacuate

Asthma

Asthma is common and causes a significant number of deaths—take it seriously. Dust, animals, pollen, cold air, work, infection, emotion and exercise can all trigger asthma attacks. Some expedition members, in some environments, may find that their asthma improves. Take steps to avoid attacks and treat asthma with appropriate medications. Those who suffer from severe asthma and have a history of frequent hospital admissions should not attempt expeditions to isolated areas.

Symptoms and signs	Treatment
☐ Short of breath, fast respiratory rate ☐ Wheeze on breathing out ☐ There may be only slight wheezing in dangerously severe attacks. Look at the casualty—if they look very unwell, they are! ☐ Inflated chest ☐ Chest infection and cough ☐ Pale, exhausted, sitting up, braced ☐ Unable to talk in sentences ☐ Peak flow <50% normal ☐ **Do not give NSAIDs or betablockers to asthmatics**	☐ Keep sitting up and give oxygen ☐ Give albuterol inhaler—4 puffs every 15 minutes ☐ If not improving, use a spacer or improvise one—inflate a plastic bag, put in 10 puffs of albuterol, get casualty to take 6 breaths ☐ Continue with albuterol until casualty improves ☐ Give prednisolone 60mg oral or, in severe attack, give hydrocortisone 100mg IV (or IM) ☐ Give antihistamine (IV or oral) ☐ Seek medical advice and evacuate

Chest infection (pneumonia)

The least serious chest infections may cause symptoms no more significant than an irritating cough; the most serious, such as pneumonia, are life-threatening.

Symptoms and signs	Treatment
□ Fever, feeling unwell □ Short of breath, fast respiratory rate □ Coughing up green sputum □ Possibly wheeze, sharp chest pain □ Crackly, coarse breath sounds	□ If very unwell (respiratory rate >40 breaths per minute, blue lips/nails), give oxygen if available □ Antibiotics for 5 days—IV if fever >102°F (>39°C), very unwell □ If not improving, seek medical advice

High blood pressure (normal <140/90, severe >160/110)

Team members with a history of high blood pressure will usually carry medication. However, if they forget or if diarrhea and vomiting prevent tablets from being absorbed, their blood pressure may be uncontrolled.

Symptoms and signs	Treatment
□ Headache □ Chest pain □ Nausea, vomiting, nose bleed □ Confusion, seizures if very severe	□ Blood pressure above 160/110 or symptoms—seek medical advice □ Give antinausea drugs and usual medication

Blood clots in the lungs (pulmonary emboli—PE) and legs (deep vein thrombosis—DVT)

Portions of blood clots that form in the leg and thigh veins (DVT's) sometimes break away (embolize) and lodge in the lungs. Large PEs can cause severe chest pain and sudden death. People at particular risk of blood clots may take warfarin and/or aspirin (or may have done so in the past). Risk factors include obesity, smoking, the oral contraceptive pill, pelvic and lower limb fractures, immobility, flying and dehydration. If a team member develops a large PE and loses consciousness, the only effective response is to attempt resuscitation (see p.28-29).

Symptoms and signs	Treatment
□ Sudden-onset shortness of breath □ Chest pain on one side □ Cough producing bloody sputum □ May be shocked or even in cardiac arrest □ Swollen, tender lower leg or thigh	□ Collapsed—assess ABC (see p.28) □ Give oxygen if available □ Pain relief: morphine 5-10mg IM □ Aspirin 300mg oral □ Seek medical advice and arrange urgent evacuation

Musculoskeletal pain

Pain originating in a specific location on the chest wall may be extreme but have no obvious cause, and the casualty may show no other signs of trauma or illness. Costochondritis (inflammation of rib/cartilage junctions) can be particularly sore.

Symptoms and signs	Treatment
□ Sudden onset at particular spot □ Pain may inhibit deep breathing □ Tenderness over the point of pain	□ Exclude other causes □ Analgesia □ May take a few days to improve

ABDOMINAL DISORDERS

If a team member has a painful and distended abdomen, take notice. Some of the disorders that cause these symptoms are serious. It is most important to recognize infection, bowel obstruction and abdominal inflammation (peritonitis) at an early stage and treat with IV hydration and antibiotics.

Constipation is a common cause of abdominal symptoms. Pay attention to proper hydration, particularly if using freeze-dried food. Angina, chest infections, urinary tract infections (see p.156), gynecological disorders (see pp.152–53) and diabetic complications (see pp.50–51) also cause abdominal pain.

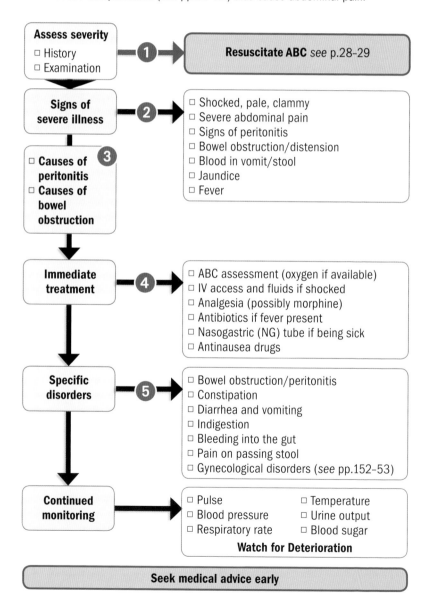

Assess severity
- □ History
- □ Examination

1 → **Resuscitate ABC** *see p.28–29*

Signs of severe illness

2 →
- □ Shocked, pale, clammy
- □ Severe abdominal pain
- □ Signs of peritonitis
- □ Bowel obstruction/distension
- □ Blood in vomit/stool
- □ Jaundice
- □ Fever

3
- □ Causes of peritonitis
- □ Causes of bowel obstruction

Immediate treatment

4 →
- □ ABC assessment (oxygen if available)
- □ IV access and fluids if shocked
- □ Analgesia (possibly morphine)
- □ Antibiotics if fever present
- □ Nasogastric (NG) tube if being sick
- □ Antinausea drugs

Specific disorders

5 →
- □ Bowel obstruction/peritonitis
- □ Constipation
- □ Diarrhea and vomiting
- □ Indigestion
- □ Bleeding into the gut
- □ Pain on passing stool
- □ Gynecological disorders (see pp.152–53)

Continued monitoring →
- □ Pulse
- □ Blood pressure
- □ Respiratory rate
- □ Temperature
- □ Urine output
- □ Blood sugar

Watch for Deterioration

Seek medical advice early

① History and examination

☐ Symptoms and signs may develop slowly; deterioration over hours or days.
☐ Previous abdominal operations may be significant—look for scars, but remember that the scars of keyhole surgery may be difficult to spot.
☐ Do not carry out a rectal or vaginal examination unless you are trained and have someone to assist you.

Important points in the history

☐ Site and severity of pain?
☐ What makes it better/worse (eating, deep breathing, antacids, vomiting)?
☐ Any nausea/vomiting/diarrhea/constipation?
☐ Women: menstrual history? Other gynecological problems? (see p.152)
☐ Previous abdominal problems?

Important points in the examination

Look
☐ Feverish, pale, jaundiced?
☐ Abdominal distension?
☐ Scars (look around the umbilicus)?
☐ Blood in vomit or stools?

Feel
☐ Pain with gentle pressing/tapping of the abdomen
☐ Any masses?

Listen
☐ Bowel sounds with stethoscope

Document vital signs, blood sugar, urine output, urine dipstick test

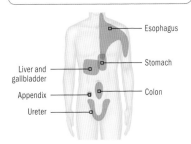

Liver and gallbladder
Appendix
Ureter
Esophagus
Stomach
Colon

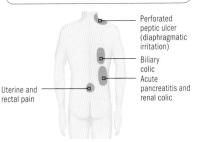

Uterine and rectal pain
Perforated peptic ulcer (diaphragmatic irritation)
Biliary colic
Acute pancreatitis and renal colic

Abdominal pain locations associated with certain organs and disorders

② Signs of severe illness

Shocked, pale, and clammy Casualty in severe pain or with low blood pressure.
Rigid/tender abdomen Casualty may have peritonitis.
Vomiting of green bile, absence of feces or flatulence (wind), abdominal distension Casualty may be suffering from a bowel obstruction.
Blood in vomit/stool Fresh or blackish blood in vomit indicates bleeding from stomach or first part of small bowel. Blood in the stool, perhaps black and very smelly, may come from the stomach, the first part of the small bowel or lower down.
Jaundice Jaundice is usually caused by liver problems; for example, gallstones.
Fever Fever signifies infection, which may result from a serious bowel problem, such as perforation, or may result from a kidney infection.

③ Causes

Causes of peritonitis

☐ Perforated bowel
☐ Appendicitis
☐ Peptic ulcer
☐ Pancreatitis
☐ Gallstones
☐ Gyne. problems

Causes of bowel obstruction

☐ Severe constipation
☐ Pancreatitis
☐ Previous surgery
☐ Twisted bowel
☐ Hernia

④ Immediate treatment

Shock Treat shock immediately. Lie the casualty down and prop the legs up above the heart. Insert an IV cannula (see pp.186–87) and give IV fluids (500ml initially—measure blood pressure). Seek medical advice immediately.

Analgesia Morphine 5–10mg IM may be used to treat severe pain. Do not use NSAIDs until you are certain there is no peptic ulceration or bleeding.

Antibiotics Administer antibiotics at an early stage if there are any signs of infection: temperature over 99.5°F (37.5°C), acute abdomen, bowel obstruction. Give IV if the casualty is vomiting or the temperature is over 102°F (39°C). Use a broad-spectrum antibiotic and metronidazole (see inside back cover).

Nasogastric (NG) tube The tube should be left open and attached to a bag, to allow the stomach to drain, reducing pain, distension and vomiting (see p.200).

Antinausea medication Administer antinausea drugs to reduce vomiting and also when using morphine. The medical kit may contain several types; seek medical advice regarding which drugs to use.

⑤ Specific conditions

Bowel obstruction/peritonitis (acute abdomen)

These are life-threatening conditions and need to be detected at an early stage. Treatment in the wilderness can be successful in containing the cause (which may well not be known) until urgent evacuation can be arranged.

Symptoms and signs	Treatment
□ Severe abdominal pain □ Pain on gentle pressing or tapping □ Rigid abdomen, possibly distended □ Fever □ Vomiting (green bile) □ Check for hernia—painful swelling in groin at top of leg □ "Tinkly" bowel sounds or silence □ Check blood sugar and chest for signs of angina, infection	□ ABC assessment if collapsed □ IV access and 500ml fluid □ Treat severe pain with morphine 5–10mg IM injection □ Antibiotics intravenously □ Antinausea drugs □ Antacid treatment (see Indigestion treatment, opposite page) □ NG tube (see p.200) and drain bag □ Watch urine output—aim for minimum 0.5ml/kg/hour

Constipation

Freeze-dried food must be properly rehydrated. Normal bowel habit varies enormously, from 3 stools per day to one stool every 3–4 days.

Symptoms and signs	Treatment
□ No stools (or very little hard stool) passed for 2–3 days longer than normal for that team member □ Cramping abdominal discomfort □ Distended abdomen if severe	□ Avoid by good hydration and high-fiber diet (aim for dilute urine) □ Treat with glycerine suppositories, stool softener (lactulose), and stimulants (bisacodyl)

Diarrhea and vomiting

The cause is usually food poisoning; rarely, an abdominal disorder. Nausea and vomiting alone may indicate motion sickness or pregnancy. Observe strict hygiene.

Symptoms and signs	Treatment
□ Vomiting or diarrhea or both □ Abdominal cramps □ Dehydration □ Vomit may be yellow, green, bloody □ Stool may be watery, black, bloody	□ Keep hydrated—rehydration drinks □ IV fluid may be needed if severely dehydrated and still vomiting □ Antinausea drugs (cyclizine) □ Antidiarrheal drugs (loperamide)

Indigestion

Indigestion is a frequent occurrence on expeditions due to a change in diet, irregular and rapidly eaten meals, stress and fatigue. The pain of severe indigestion may be mistaken for a heart attack (and vice versa).

Symptoms and signs	Treatment
□ Pain over upper part of abdomen or in chest □ Pain may be burning or gripping □ Stomach acid may reflux into mouth	□ Simple antacids □ Medications that reduce acid in stomach (ranitidine, lansoprazole)

Bleeding into the gut

The likely causes of blood in vomit are a bleeding stomach or a duodenal ulcer. Blood in or on stool is most likely to have come from bleeding piles or from another part of the lower bowel. Treatment is limited and the casualty should be evacuated.

Symptoms and signs	Treatment
□ Vomit containing fresh blood or blood like coffee grounds □ Fresh blood on the surface of the stool or tarry black stool (melena) □ Shock may develop □ Inspect around anus if blood on stool or on toilet paper □ History of peptic ulcer disease	□ IV access and 500ml fluid if shocked—seek medical advice □ Medications that reduce acid in stomach (ranitidine, lansoprazole); use type that is absorbed in the mouth □ Monitor urine output—aim for minimum 0.5ml/hour/kg □ Seek medical advice and evacuate

Pain on passing stool

This is very unpleasant, can be excruciating and may result in avoidance of passing stool and serious constipation. Simple treatments can be effective.

Symptoms and signs	Treatment
□ Pain on passing stool, worse with hard-formed stool □ Traces of blood on the stool □ Piles may come out of anus □ An anal fissure may be visible	□ Keep hydrated to keep stool soft □ Avoid constipation (see p.150) □ Analgesia—lidocaine gel rubbed up inside the anus before passing stool may help

GYNECOLOGICAL DISORDERS

The female reproductive organs may cause symptoms due to normal functions (menstruation, pregnancy) or as a result of disease (infection).

Performing an examination of the genital area requires sensitivity and discretion. Unless you are trained and experienced, internal examination of the vagina will probably not be useful. Seek medical advice if you are not sure whether to proceed.

Menstruation and contraception

Some women may choose to control or even suppress their menstrual cycle completely. Consultation with a doctor six months before a long expedition will allow time for new methods to be tried and changed if necessary. Options for long-term contraception and suppression of menstruation include:

Combined oral contraception ("the pill") Placebo week is eliminated. When each pack of 21 pills is finished, a new set of active pills is started immediately.

Depot injection Injections provide contraception for three months. Spotting may occur during the first three-month treatment, followed by menstruation suppression.

Implant Contraceptive implants provide contraception for up to three years and can be removed at any time. Spotting may occur in the first three months. Menstruation will be suppressed after that.

Intrauterine (IU) contraceptive device IU devices are inserted into the uterus, providing contraception immediately and reducing menstrual bleeding after three to six months.

Pregnancy

The two complications of most concern are miscarriage and ectopic pregnancy (see p.153). Symptoms of severe abdominal pain and heavy bleeding from the vagina should be investigated immediately. Pregnancy can exacerbate nausea, such as motion sickness, but seek medical advice before giving any antinausea medication.

History and examination

- Be diplomatic and respect confidentiality.
- Gynecological disorders should be among the causes considered if a female team member suffers an acute abdomen and collapse.
- Do not perform a vaginal examination unless you are trained to do so.
- Is there a history of gynecological problems?
- Test for pregnancy at an early stage, if you have a testing kit. These tests are easy and provide immediate results.

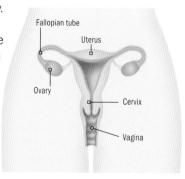

Fallopian tube

Uterus

Ovary

Cervix

Vagina

Female reproductive organs

Important points in the history	Important points in the examination

☐ Pelvic or abdominal pain?
☐ Possibility of pregnancy?
☐ Bleeding or discharge from vagina?
☐ Change to menstrual cycle
  – Absent or bleeding mid-cycle?
  – More blood than normal/pain?
☐ Pain and frequency passing urine?
☐ Method of contraception?
☐ Number and outcome of any
  previous pregnancies?
	Look
	☐ Pale, in pain, shocked, feverish?
	☐ Check discharge (on a pad)
	Feel
	☐ Abdomen for tenderness and
	  rigidity, swelling arising out of pelvis
	Listen
	☐ Bowel sounds through stethoscope
	Document vital signs, pregnancy
	test, urine dipstick test

Specific symptoms/conditions

Vaginal bleeding

Stress, fatigue, change of contraception and pregnancy can all interrupt the normal menstrual cycle. Unexpected bleeding may indicates miscarriage, ectopic pregnancy, intercourse or inflammation. Seek medical advice.

Symptoms and signs	Treatment
☐ Signs of shock—pale, sweaty, cold ☐ Tender abdomen ☐ Try to quantify blood loss—clots? ☐ Pregnancy test and urine dipstick	☐ Treat shock with IV fluids ☐ Analgesia ☐ Oxytocin may reduce bleeding in miscarriage

Ectopic pregnancy

This occurs when the fertilized egg implants in the fallopian tube before arriving at the uterus. As the embryo grows, it causes pain and may eventually rupture the tube, causing serious bleeding into the abdomen. Bleeding from the vagina may be minor.

Symptoms and signs	Treatment

☐ Signs of shock—pale, sweaty, cold
☐ Severe abdominal pain (one-sided)
☐ Usually happens around week 6–8
  after last period
☐ Pregnancy test usually positive
	☐ Treat shock—lie down/legs raised
	☐ IV fluids—give 1L and seek
	  medical advice
	☐ Analgesia
	☐ Arrange urgent evacuation

Discharge and infection

Infection may be indicated by offensive green, yellow or watery discharge, vaginal discomfort or pain on passing urine. A foul, black discharge may be caused by a forgotten tampon. The discharge should settle once the tampon is removed, but antibiotics may be required if the casualty is feverish and unwell.

Symptoms and signs	Treatment

☐ Change in color/amount of discharge
☐ Fever, feeling unwell, frequency
  of urination
☐ Abdominal pain or discomfort
	☐ If discharge is thick, white: treat
	  for thrush (clotrimazole pessary)
	☐ Treat infections with erythromycin
	  and metronidazole

URINARY, KIDNEY AND GENITAL DISORDERS

Good hygiene is more difficult to maintain on expeditions, so the risk of infection is increased. Disorders of the urinary system and genitals should be treated promptly.

Infections of the urinary tract are common, particularly in women, whose anatomy may allow bacteria to collect more readily. Infections of both male and female genitalia can cause extreme discomfort. It is sensible to practice safe sex and use condoms to avoid sexually transmitted infections. Kidney infections may make the casualty very unwell, causing shock and a high fever. If you suspect a kidney infection, seek medical advice.

Injury, torsion and infection of the male testes are all extremely painful. Torsion of the testes is an emergency. Surgery should take place within 6–12 hours if possible. Examination of this area calls for discretion and sensitivity. If you are uncertain about any aspect of examination, seek medical advice.

Passing blood

A reasonably small amount of blood can cause the urine to look completely red. This can be a frightening symptom, so reassure the casualty. They are unlikely to lose a significant amount of blood in the urine or go into shock. Administer treatment appropriate to the likely cause. Note, however, that bleeding in the urine over a number of days may cause the casualty to become anemic, which will manifest as paleness, lethargy and malaise. If you suspect anemia, seek medical advice and arrange urgent evacuation.

Causes of blood in the urine
- Infection of the urinary tract—see p.156
- Renal stones—see p.157
- Vaginal bleeding coloring the urine
- Trauma (such as pelvic fracture, see pp.116–17, or as a result of inserting a urinary catheter), which should settle
- Use of medications such as warfarin, aspirin, clopidogrel—seek medical advice if this is the case
- Other diseases of the kidneys and renal tract—refer to a doctor when possible
- Red coloration of the urine may be caused by drugs (rifampin) and foods such as beets (in large quantities)

History and examination

- Be diplomatic and respect confidentiality.
- Do not perform a vaginal or rectal examination unless trained to do so.
- If there is genital infection, sexual partners may also be infected. This may cause embarrassment, but the problem must be dealt with. Be as sensitive as possible.

Important points in the history	Important points in the examination
□ Site and severity of pain (including testicles, scrotum and abdomen) □ Amount and color of discharge □ Pain and frequency passing urine □ Color and smell of urine □ Any sores, swellings or ulcers on genitals or around anus □ Sexual contacts □ Test urine with dipstick □ Pregnancy test for women	**Look** □ Appearance (pale, in pain, feverish, shocked) □ Inflammation, sores, lumps, discharge □ Swollen, reddish-blue scrotum **Feel** □ Lower abdomen for tender or swollen bladder □ Flanks for tenderness over kidney □ Scrotum and testicles for swelling and tenderness

Specific conditions

Urinary retention

On an expedition, the most likely causes of urinary retention are infection, prostatism in older men, pelvic or genitalia trauma, blood clot in the bladder, drugs (antihistamines and some anti-depressants) or loss of consciousness, if prolonged. To treat, pass a catheter into the bladder through the urethra (*see* p.201). Do not try to pass a catheter if there is blood in the urine following trauma. The other option—inserting a suprapubic catheter (*see* p.202)—is a specialized procedure and you must seek medical advice for guidance.

Symptoms and signs	Treatment
□ Inability to pass urine despite urge to do so □ Fullness and tender lower abdomen □ History of trauma □ Signs of infection	□ Seek medical advice first before attempting to insert a catheter—it might make matters worse □ A suprapubic catheter may be required (*see* p.202) □ Leave catheter in and evacuate

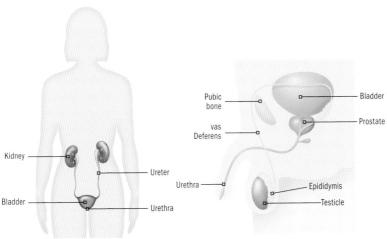

Female urinary tract

Kidney

Ureter

Bladder

Urethra

Male urinary tract

Pubic bone

vas Deferens

Urethra

Bladder

Prostate

Epididymis

Testicle

Scrotal pain/testicular torsion

Testicular torsion, or twisting, stops blood supply to the testis, resulting in sudden, extreme pain and even vomiting. If the twisting is not reversed swiflty (possibly within 6 hours), the testis will die. This reversal would normally be performed surgically, but manual untwisting may be attempted in the wilderness under medical guidance. Note, however, that the manual method is not always successful.

Symptoms and signs	Treatment
□ Sudden, severe testicular pain □ Very tender testis on gentle palpation □ Scrotum may become red, swollen □ No history of trauma—pain may cause the casualty to wake	□ Strong analgesia and antinausea medication □ Seek medical advice and attempt manual untwisting □ Evacuate urgently whether successful or not

Manual untwisting of a torted testis
□ Position the casualty lying down with the scrotum elevated
□ Gently but firmly hold affected testis in fingers and rotate toward the inner thigh on that side (that is; rotate his right testis anticlockwise, as you look at it, and his left testis clockwise). These are the directions that work most often.
□ Relief of pain will be immediate, but more than one turn may be necessary
□ Try rotating in the opposite direction if pain increases

Scrotal pain/epididymitis

Inflammation usually affects either part or the whole of one testis only. It is most often caused by infection, which may be sexually transmitted. Inflammation must not be confused with testicular torsion—seek medical advice if necessary.

Symptoms and signs	Treatment
□ Gradual-onset pain from one testis □ Scrotum may become red, swollen □ Fever, and pain passing urine □ Urine dipstick may show blood and protein in the urine	□ Pain may be relieved by lying down and gently elevating scrotum (for example, on a rolled-up towel) □ Analgesia □ Antibiotics if signs of infection

Urinary tract infection

Infection may occur in various parts of the urinary tract, from the urethra to the kidney. Women are particularly susceptible. Kidney infections may progress to high fever, sepsis and shock.

Symptoms and signs	Treatment
□ Fever □ Kidney infections—very unwell, possibly shocked, flank pain □ Pain and frequency on passing urine □ Urine dipstick—positive for protein, blood, white cells, nitrites	□ If in shock—IV access/fluid and seek medical advice □ Analgesia □ Antibiotics (IV if very unwell) □ Keep hydrated—aim for dilute urine

Kidney (renal) stones

Physical exertion and dehydration in a hot climate may cause stones to form in the kidney. As they are passed, severe pain extends from the flank down to the groin. Complications include obstruction, if stones become lodged in the ureter or bladder, and infection. Stones and infection may cause blood in the urine, turning it reddish.

Symptoms and signs	Treatment
□ Sudden severe pain in one flank □ Nausea and vomiting, fever □ Dipstick testing may show blood, protein, nitrites and white cells	□ Keep well hydrated □ Analgesia—acetaminophen, NSAIDs □ Antibiotics if feverish □ Seek medical advice if symptoms do not improve

Sexually transmitted diseases (STDs)

Any STD is significant, whether very serious (syphilis, HIV) or simple to treat (chlamydia, gonorrhea). Sexual contacts will need to be traced and treated, despite the potential embarrassment. Avoid all sexual contact (including oral contact) if an STD is suspected.

Symptoms and signs	Treatment
□ Green, offensive discharge from penis or vagina □ Pain passing urine, sores on genitals	□ Cause will probably not be identified in the wilderness □ Antibiotics (such as ciprofloxacin)

Genital sores and lumps

Ulcers, blisters and sores are usually the result of infection, possibly an STD. Herpes causes numerous, painful blisters and ulcers. A mild tingling will usually occur first—apply acyclovir cream at this stage. Syphilis is likely to cause single, painless, hard-edged and clean ulcers. Swellings and abscesses (sometimes in the labia) may be caused by bacterial infection; these may discharge without treatment but sometimes need antibiotics and even surgery. Genital warts or the small white lumps caused by molluscum contagiosum do not require urgent treatment, but avoid sexual contact, and do not share towels or bed linen.

Foreskin problems

If the foreskin is pulled back over the head of the penis and not put back again, it may become very swollen. If infection develops, due to an STD or poor personal hygiene, the area under the foreskin may become inflamed.

Symptoms and signs	Treatment
□ Swollen, retracted foreskin—may be very enlarged □ Inflammation and whitish discharge under foreskin. There may be pain on passing urine	□ Lidocaine gel on foreskin for pain, then gentle, long squeeze to reduce swelling. Return foreskin to usual position □ Infection—thorough, regular washing under foreskin. Clotrimazole cream/antibiotics if not improving/severe

INFECTIOUS DISEASES

Travel to different areas of the world brings expedition members into contact with new, potentially disease-causing organisms against which they may have no natural immunity. For this reason, infection—usually of the gut or skin—is one of the most common medical problems affecting expeditions.

The danger from infection is generally low, but some infections may be life-threatening. Even common infective problems, such as food poisoning and diarrhea, are unpleasant, inconvenient and draining. In the wilderness, infection can also increase the risks of other problems such as dehydration, hypothermia, injury and altitude sickness. Learn about any specific risks in the area you will be visiting and encourage all expedition members to take personal responsibility; they should disclose existing illnesses and maintain good hygiene.

Vehicles of infection

Food and milk Undercooked/untreated food and milk carry high risk (*see* p.73).
Water To minimize contamination, make sure all water is clean or treated before putting it in water bottles. Clean your teeth in treated water (*see* p.75–76).
Clothing and bedding Micro-organisms and larger pests may inhabit clothes and sleeping bags. Clean as regularly as possible, and disinfect at the beginning and end of an expedition.
Expedition members Team members may be harboring infections such as food poisoning, sexually transmitted diseases or chronic infectious diseases, including hepatitis or human immunodeficiency virus. All members should declare any infections before the start of the expedition. If the degree of risk is accurately known, control measures can be put in place.
Animals Insects are common vehicles of infection, especially in tropical and sub-tropical areas. In particular mosquitoes, ticks, worms and sand flies transmit serious diseases. Take rigorous preventative measures to prevent bites (*see* p.82).

Preparation

Knowledge of area Government agencies, local agencies and travel guides can provide information on prevalent diseases in the area. This knowledge will help in compiling an appropriate medical kit and in making provisional diagnoses in the field. Forewarned is forearmed.
Vaccinations Either vaccinations or boosters are recommended before travel to most countries. A certificate of yellow fever immunization is needed for entry into some countries. *See* p.222 for guidance on specific vaccination requirements.
Medical kit Your kit should take into account any infections you are likely to encounter. For instance, extra ciprofloxacin (an antibiotic used for treating gut infections) may be appropriate for expeditions to the Indian sub-continent. Special medications may be required for malarial areas and those where rabies is endemic.
Team members The previous medical history of a team member may significantly increase the risk of serious illness when traveling to areas where infection is prevalent. Any chronic disease or medication that increases susceptibility to infection may prohibit inclusion of that team member on the expedition.

Prevention

Behavior If you know you have a transmissible disease, do not go on an expedition into the wilderness without making a full disclosure beforehand.

Personal hygiene Maintain a high level of personal hygiene at all times and be scrupulously clean when cooking.

Food and drink Take rigorous precautions at all times (*see* p.73–76).

Anti-bite measures Precautions such as permethrin-impregnated mosquito nets, long trousers, long-sleeved shirts and insect repellent may be required in some areas and certainly when traveling to areas where mosquitoes are common.

Contamination Contact with bodily fluids, particularly blood, should be avoided. Wear gloves, eye protection and masks when cleaning and flushing wounds.

Antimalarial drugs Always use antimalarials for prevention when traveling to endemic malarial areas. Seek advice for the specific area as resistance is possible.

Early antibiotics When in the remote wilderness, it is advisable to treat possible infections at an early stage to avoid deterioration, the onset of sepsis and shock.

Diagnosis in the wilderness

A definitive diagnosis of an infection's cause is unlikely in the field, but a provisional diagnosis may help you to target treatment and assess the need for evacuation.

Location Some infectious diseases are geographically constrained (yellow fever for example, only occurs in Latin America and equatorial Africa), so can be eliminated from the list of possible diagnoses outside these areas.

Local knowledge Local travel guides and medics may have more detailed knowledge of the distribution of a particular infectious disease (for example, some diseases only occur on flood plains and not at higher altitudes).

Vaccination history A vaccine against an infectious disease will significantly reduce risk, but no vaccine reduces the risk of infection to zero.

Course of disease Diseases have incubation periods before symptoms become evident. For instance, malaria can only become symptomatic at least seven days after entering an endemic area for the first time.

Symptoms The developing symptoms may well give a clue to possible diagnosis. A team member who develops a rash is very unlikely to have malaria and one that develops an expanding red circle (erythema migrans) around a tick bite is likely to have Lyme disease.

Response to treatment Failure to respond casts doubt on the diagnosis.

Treatment

Treatment is aimed at controlling the infection and preventing transmission.

Isolation Avoid using the same bedding, towels and clothes to reduce transmission risk. If a team member has immunity to a disease, such as chickenpox, they alone should attend to the casualty.

Hygiene Cleanliness is vital to prevent infection spreading. Gut infections may spread rapidly if the cook is infected and is less than fastidious with hygiene.

Medications After all precautions have been taken, medications such as antibiotics are the final measure. In general, signs of infection should be treated more readily in the wilderness, because the consequences of leaving the infection untreated are more serious.

Nutrition and hydration Proper nutrition and hydration will aid the immune system and improve recovery. For various methods of hydration, *see* p.184–185.

Infections	Organism	Location	Transmission	Symptoms and Signs	Treatment	Vaccine
African trypanosomiasis (sleeping sickness)	Protozoan parasite	Eastern, western, and central Africa	Tsetse fly	Painful bite, fever, headache, joint pains, then very enlarged (△) lymph nodes, particularly back of neck, shoulders. Increasing malaise, confusion, fatigue.	Avoid bites, cover up, use repellent and permethrin netting. Pentamidine, suramin or eflornithine initially. Melarprosole, eflornithine, nifurtimox for nervous system involvement.	No
Chagas disease (American trypansomiasis)	Protozoan parasite	North, Central, South America	Triatomine bugs, açaí fruit juice, cane sugar juice, blood transfusions	Incubation 1-2 weeks. Sore around bite, swollen eyelid. Acute stage: fever, malaise. △ lymph glands, △ liver and spleen. Chronic stage: heart problems, △ oesophagus/colon	At night; avoid bug bites, cover up, use permethrin netting. Avoid uncooked food. Treat to control, not cure. Benznidazole[2] 5-7mg/kg/day 3 divided doses oral for 1-4 months	No (under development)
Dengue fever	Virus	Southeast Asia, South America, Caribbean	Mosquito	Fever, headache, aches, blotchy rash that blanches, rarely bleeding from nose and gut, shock	Support symptoms, control fever and hydrate. Evacuate if severe and bleeding. Avoid mosquitos	No
Hepatitis A	Virus	Mostly developing countries	Fecal-oral route (unwashed food)	Fever, chills, vomiting, fatigue, jaundice, pale stool, dark urine	Support symptoms, hydrate, isolate until improvement, no alcohol	Yes
Infestations	Lice, fleas and mites (scabies), and ticks	Widespread	Clothes, bedding, sexual contact, animals (domestic pets and wild)	Itching of head, groin, skin, infected bites; scabies—long burrows between fingers, wrists. May transmit other diseases: typhus, Lyme disease, plague, tick-borne encephalitis (TBE)	Malathion orally for scabies and lice. Antihistamine for itch. Treat with long-acting insecticide for fleas. Remove ticks with tweezers. Watch for other symptoms of disease	No
Japanese B encephalitis	Virus	Widespread in Asia, occasionally in north Australia	Mosquito	Headache, lethargy, fever, confusion, possibly tremors and seizures, reduced consciousness	Avoid mosquito bites. No direct treatment. Supportive, hydration, isolation. Seek medical advice and evacuate urgently	Yes
Leishmaniasis —Cutaneous —Visceral (Kala azar)	Protozoan parasite	Worldwide— sub-tropical and tropical countries	Sand flies	C: incubation days–weeks. Painless prominent skin lesion. May heal with scars. V: incubation weeks–years. Fever, △ liver/spleen, skin nodules later	Avoid bites, wear sensible clothing, use repellents, permethrin-treated netting. Seek advice for drug treatment. C: sodium stibogluconate, pentamidine, itraconazole. V: miltefosine, amphoteracin B	No
Leptospirosis (Weil's disease)	Spirochete bacterium	Worldwide	Infected animal urine (e.g. rats, bats, amphibians, birds)—in water,	Incubation 2-20 days. Headache, myalgia, high fever, jaundice, blood in urine, renal failure	Avoid prolonged immersion in fresh water, particularly with open sores, wounds. Prevent: doxycycline 200–250mg 1 x weekly. Treat: doxycycline 100mg 2 x p/d for 1 week	No

Disease	Cause	Region	Transmission	Symptoms	Treatment	Vaccine
Lyme disease	Bacterium	North America, Europe	Ticks	Incubation 7-10 days. Expanding red circle around bite (Erythema migrans), swollen lymph nodes in region, fever, fatigue, arthralgia, myalgia, arthritis. Nerve/heart problems may occur later	Remove ticks with tweezers if found. Inspect body daily in high-risk areas. Treat early with doxycycline 100mg 2 x p/d or amoxicillin 500mg 4 x p/d for 2–4 weeks	No
Malaria	Protozoa	Africa, Americas, Asia, southern Europe	Mosquito	Incubation 7 days–months. High fever daily, sweating, headache, muscle aches, diarrhea, jaundice, shock, seizures, coma, heart failure	If symptoms, seek medical advice and evacuate urgently. Avoid mosquito bites. Consider quinine, mefloquine	No. Protective drugs recommended. Seek advice
Meningitis, meningococcal septicemia	Bacterium	Widespread in close communities	Air-borne droplet spread, direct contact	Fever, headache, photophobia, neck ache, non-blanching rash (sepsis), shock, coma	Urgent antibiotics (cefotaxime, benzyl penicillin, intravenous). Analgesia, IV fluids for shock. Seek medical advice and evacuate	Yes for some causes
Onchocerciasis (river blindness)	Filarial worms	Tropical Africa, Yemen, Saudi Arabia, South America (central/north)	Black flies	Skin nodules and itchy rash, △ lymph glands, eye disease leading to blindness. Symptoms may occur over a year after exposure.	Destroy black fly larvae. Wear protective clothing, repellents and avoid infected areas. Ivermectin 150µg/kg 1–2 doses p/year; rarely surgical removal/worms; doxycycline may help	No
Rabies	Virus	Widespread	Bite/saliva from rabid animal: dog, cat, bat, cow, sheep etc. Any bite by sick-looking dog—assume rabies.	Incubation period 2–12 months or more. Itching at site of bite, headache, fever, confusion, hallucinations, hydrophobia–spasm of throat when attempting to drink, loss of consciousness	Scrub wound with antiseptic. Antibiotics and tetanus for other infections. Previous vaccine: 2 boosters on days 0 and 7. No previous vaccine: post-exposure vaccine course and 1 dose rabies immune globulin. Seek medical advice and evacuate	Yes
Schistosomiasis (bilharzia)	Schistosoma flukes	Brasil, Venezuela, Middle East, India, Far East, China	Fluke larvae from snails penetrate human skin in water	Early stage:itch, raised blotchy skin rash, fever, cough, abdominal pain, diarrhea, fatigue. Later: △ liver and spleen, genital sores, liver/renal failure	Prevent: avoid bathing in known infected water. Early suspicion, especially if others in team become infected. Treat: single dose praziquantel yearly	No (under development)

Continued overleaf

INFECTIOUS DISEASES

161

* Not currently commercially available in the US or Canada. Contact the Centers for Disease Control and Prevention (CDC).

Continued

Infections	Organism	Location	Transmission	Symptoms and Signs	Treatment	Vaccine
Tick-borne encephalitis	Virus	Europe, Asia	Ticks, untreated dairy products	Flu-like illness initially, later increased fever, meningitis, decrease in consciousness	No specific treatment. Supportive, control fever, hydration. Seek medical advice and evacuate	Yes
Typhoid/paratyphoid	Bacterium	Widespread (common in Asia)	Fecal-oral route (unwashed food)	Incubation 8–21 days. Fever, headache, cough, abdominal pain, diarrhea/constipation, blanching rash on abdomen, gut bleed, shock	Isolate; strict hygiene to prevent spread; antibiotics—ciprofloxacin. Seek medical advice (symptoms similar to malaria) and evacuate	Yes
Typhus, rocky mountain spotted fever (RMSF), scrub typhus, African tick fever	Rickettsial bacterium	Widespread	Ticks, mites, fleas	Incubation 2–14 days. Fever, chills, headache, photophobia, nausea, abdominal pain, myalgia, rash on hands and feet after 2–5 days. RMSF may progress to seizures, coma	Remove ticks with tweezers if found. Inspect body daily in high-risk areas. Treat early with doxycycline 200mg or chloramphenicol 50mg/kg in 4 divided doses p/d for 5 days or for 2 days after fever subsides. May relapse	No
Worm infections	Various worms	Americas, Asia, Africa	Infected water, lakes, rivers; fecal-oral route	Worms seen in feces and vomit. Skin rashes and anal itching at night. Some worms cause serious illness	Do not bathe in infected water. Strict hygiene. For known infections—mebendazole	No
Yellow fever	Virus	Africa, South America	Mosquito	Incubation 3–7 days. Headache, fever, chills, aches, vomiting, stomach pain, jaundice, gut bleeding, shock	No direct treatment. Support symptoms, treat shock, and evacuate urgently	Yes, mandatory in some countries

MOTION SICKNESS

Long vehicle journeys on unpaved roads, light aircraft flights (particularly over hot terrain) and prolonged voyages at sea or on large inland waterways are all potent triggers of motion sickness. This may leave a team member in a debilitated condition at very start of the expedition.

Assess the extent of motion sickness in all expedition members and institute effective management before departing. In more than 90 percent of people, motion sickness can be prevented or at least controlled effectively. Once motion sickness has become established, frequent reassessment of the situation and appropriate action will, in the vast majority of cases, prevent escalation.

Symptoms and signs of motion sickness

Stomach	Brain
□ Loss of appetite	□ Pallor and sweating
□ Fullness of stomach	□ Dizziness, drowsiness
□ Nausea	□ Yawning, excessive breathing
□ Vomiting/retching	□ Headache, malaise
□ Occasional blood in vomit	□ Dry mouth or increase in saliva

Prevention

□ Avoid heavy meals, alcohol and recreational drugs before setting off.
□ **Start anti-sickness remedies 12–24 hours before departure**; suitable drugs should be established before an extended journey.
□ If journeying by boat, sleep on board the night before departure if possible and get a good night's rest.
□ Dress appropriately: keep adequately warm and dry, not cold or over warm.
□ Keep occupied but do not read in a vehicle; on a boat, do not go below to do chart work or cook.
□ Get as much fresh air as you can; keep a window open in a vehicle. Fix your gaze on land, clouds, stars or the horizon, which provide a stable reference point. Drive or helm if possible.
□ Keep hydrated, taking small amounts of water (or sugary drink) and small frequent snacks, even if continuing to be sick. There will be some benefit.
□ Finally, be positive and believe in a rapid recovery.

Duties of the non-sick

Expedition members who are resistant to sickness may have to take on the duties of those who are ill. Sufferers may be uncoordinated and, in severe cases, disorientated. Somebody should be responsible for them at all times (ensuring they do not fall over the side while vomiting on a boat, for example) and supply a bucket, wet wipes, a water bottle and dry cookies. Sick members may be encouraged to drive or helm, as the distraction of performing a continual task, together with fixing on stationary objects, will reduce the feeling of nausea.

Treatment

Motion sickness medications work on a variety of chemical pathways in the brain and gut, and each produces a slightly different effect. Each person will find a particular medication (or combination of medications) that works best for them.

The most commonly used medications are included in the table below. Start at the top of the table until you find one that is acceptable. Do not combine medications that have the same action. Do not combine with prescription medication without consulting the family doctor, as they might interact.

Medication	Route	Dose	Way it works	Notes
Meclizine	Oral	12.5mg twice a day	Antihistamine	May cause drowsiness, fatigue, blurred vision, dry nose, throat or mouth
Domperidone (not available in U.S.A.)	Oral	10–20mg every 6h	Peripheral antidopamine	Well tolerated, nonsedating. Convert from suppositories once vomiting stops
	Suppository	30mg every 6h (orally when able)		
Prochlorperazine	Oral	10mg every 6h	Central antidopamine	Some sedative properties, dry mouth, rarely causes abnormal movements, tremor and restlessness
	Under tongue	3mg every 6h		
	IM injection	12.5mg injection, then oral therapy 6h later		
Scopolamine	Patch behind ear	Replace patch every 72h, on the opposite side	Anticholinergic	Sedative effects, dry mouth; rarely, difficulty passing urine. Take care with patch as contamination will dilate pupil and blur vision. Wash hands after use.
	Oral	0.3mg every 8h		
Ondansetron	Oral	4–8mg every 8h	Antiserotonin	Nonsedating, occasional constiptation
	Under tongue	4–8mg every 8h		
Cyclizine	Oral	50mg every 8h	Antihistamine	Slight sedation only. Painful injection
	IM injection	50mg every 8h		
Promethazine	Oral	25mg every 6–8h	Antihistamine	Significant sedation, which may be an advantage. Dry mouth; rarely, difficulty passing urine

Alternative treatments

Some alternative treatments may work well for some crew. Wrist bands can provide acupressure or electrical pulses over the neiguan (P6) acupuncture point. Ginger root (1g every 8 hours) may also be effective.

SKIN DISORDERS

Sun, heat, cold, damp, saltwater and abrasion can all damage the skin. Secondary bacterial and other infections make skin damage much worse and may cause systemic illness. The effects of heat and cold on the skin are covered on pp.62–65 and 66–69.

Protection measures

Reduce time of sun exposure Always keep in mind how long you have been in the sun. Be particularly aware of exposure around sand, sea or snow, as there is increased reflection of sunlight.

Protective clothing when exposed Wear a wide-brimmed hat, long sleeves and long pants. Gloves may be necessary to protect the back of the hands.

Routine sunscreen Use physical screens such as zinc or titanium oxide-based creams or high factor chemical screens (>SPF 15) containing para-aminobenzoic acid or cinnamates. Water-resistant agents are ideal.

Sunglasses Make sure your sunglasses are robust and have protection at the sides. Take extras.

Gloves Wear gloves to reduce abrasion and contact with hazardous substances from plants and animals. Take extras.

Footwear Wear appropriate footwear, particularly in areas where you might encounter poisonous animals, such as snakes and scorpions, and in tropical areas. Check your footwear for unwelcome visitors every morning.

Regular moisturizer Apply to hands and feet regularly and frequently. This is not a "soft" thing to do, but wise. Fingers, toes and heels may crack at altitude or in the extreme cold, allowing secondary infection.

Personal hygiene Take responsibility for your own hygiene. Pay particular attention to the feet and groin, which are areas prone to fungal infections. Dry as thoroughly as possible and keep all parts aired.

Clothing Make sure your clothes and bedding are free of any infestations such as fleas before setting off on the expedition. Change or clean your own gear as often as practical.

Infections Treat early if there are signs of infection, including inflammation, rash, itching, spots, boils or bites.

Specific Conditions

Seek medical advice if the condition is non-healing after a few days of treatment.

Itchy skin (eczema, dermatitis, allergy)

Itching may be caused by an ongoing condition, such as eczema, or by contact with substances causing inflammation of the skin (dermatitis).

Symptoms and signs	Treatment
□ Onset of itch, which may be associated with a rash, cracked skin, contact with known irritant	□ Remove substance if known
	□ Antihistamine, aqueous creams, emollients
□ Do not scratch—damages the skin and may cause secondary infection	□ Steroid cream (hydrocortisone 1%) may be required

Sunburn

Wind, reflected UV light and lack of shade all increase the risk of severe sunburn.

Symptoms and signs	Treatment
□ Red, painful skin on exposed parts □ Dehydration, malaise, nausea □ Casualty feels chilly but skin is hot □ Blisters and swelling if severe	□ Keep hydrated and in the shade □ Acetaminophen and NSAIDs □ Hydrocortisone 1% cream may help □ Do not burst blisters

Rashes

Infection, allergic reactions and abrasive conditions are common causes of rashes of varying types. A non-blanching rash may indicate meningitis (see p.133).

Symptoms and signs	Treatment
□ Red, raised, blotchy, itchy lumps (hives)—likely to be allergic reaction □ Rashes with spreading or pus-exuding sores may be infective □ Rash in armpits and on waist, chest, back may be prickly heat (see p.67)	□ Look for source of allergy and treat accordingly (see pp.48-49) □ Infection may be bacterial, viral, or fungal (see below) □ Heat rash—keep area dry and clean. Calamine or hydrocortisone cream

Skin infections

Impetigo in particular can spread rapidly through a team in close living quarters.

Symptoms and signs	Treatment
Viral (shingles/herpes)—very painful blisters that erupt and crust, usually in one area. Patient may be unwell prior to rash **Bacterial** □ Impetigo—crusting blisters that spread in patches; itchy, red, painful □ Cellulitis—painful, red, spreading from a wound site or blisters □ Fungal—generally in groin or between toes. Reddish with raised margin, spreading outward, cracking skin	**Shingles** Analgesia, antibiotics only if blisters become infected **Impetigo** Strict hygiene (no sharing towels etc). Antibiotics: dicloxacillin and mupirocin cream. Seek medical advice if not improving after 3 days **Cellulitis** Antibiotics: amoxicillin + clavulanate. Seek medical advice if it does not improve after 3 days or rapidly spreads **Fungal infection** Miconazole cream for 10 days. Keep clean and dry

Tropical ulcers, abscesses and boils

Tropical ulcers start from a scratch or wound on the shin. A pustule forms then discharges days later, forming a painful, hard-edged ulcer. Seek medical input.

Symptoms and signs	Treatment
□ **Tropical ulcers**—non-healing ulcer, painful, hard, under-eroded edge □ **Abscesses and boils**—usually a bacterial infection in or under the skin. Painful until drained. May cause a spreading skin infection (cellulitis). Abscesses on the buttocks, breast, and peri-anal area require specialist treatment.	□ **Tropical ulcers**—Antibiotics: Amoxicillin & clavulanate or possibly metronidazole—seek medical advice when possible for further treatment □ **Abscesses and boils**—May point and drain on their own, otherwise lance (see p.197). Treat with amoxicillin & clavulanate

FOOT BLISTERS

Blisters can quickly ruin enjoyment of trekking and may even become disabling. As with most problems, prevention is the best strategy. Failing that, early detection of "hot spots" or small blisters is vital. Treatment may then prevent deterioration.

Cause

□ Friction between skin and sock
□ Build-up of moisture in boot

▼

□ Increased heat energy in skin
□ Increased moisture softens skin

▼

□ Friction causes breakdown of softened skin layers

▼

□ Fluid accumulates between split layers

BLISTER FORMATION

□ Usually contain clear lymph fluid
□ Occasionally contain blood (if there is trauma) or pus (if there is infection)

Prevention

The key to prevention is to reduce friction on the skin and moisture in the boot.
□ Wear well-fitting boots with no tight points and adequate toe room.
□ Use breathable (e.g. Gortex™-lined) boots to avoid moisture build-up.
□ Keep interior of boots free from sand/gravel etc. that may cause friction.
□ Ensure laces are at correct tension to reduce movement of foot within boot, without causing compression/restriction.
□ Wear "ragg" or loop-stitch socks with good moisture wicking ability.
□ Alternate pairs of socks to keep as dry as possible.
□ Liner socks may reduce skin friction.
□ Cool and dry feet at any opportunity.
□ Use deodorant stick or petroleum jelly to lubricate friction points or hot spots—will require frequent reapplication but is effective.

Treatment

Intervene as soon as hot spots appear—they will turn into blisters if not treated.
□ If blister is large and tense with fluid, puncture and drain fluid under sterile conditions. Do not de-roof blister, but apply dressing as below.
□ Small blisters and hot spots: apply a thick dressing (e.g. foam mattress or padding) with a hole the size of the blister cut in the middle. Tape firmly in place.
□ De-roofed blisters: burst blisters, clean with antiseptic (dry iodine spray) then dress with absorbable dressing ("second skin"). These can stay in place for a few days before change is required.
□ Hot spots or small blisters: tape over with duct tape or similar to reduce friction.
□ Duct tape is cheap and very effective for lining the inside of boots, or applying directly to the skin.
□ Monitor de-roofed/burst blisters for infection and treat immediately.

OVERDOSES AND POISONING

Prescription drugs and recreational substances can both cause deliberate or accidental overdose. Carbon monoxide is a risk in poorly ventilated tents and shelters when using gas stoves or heating. Prolonged engine use in vehicles also carries risk. Chlorine is another potential poison, particularly on boats if the battery bank floods.

If a team member takes an overdose, it is vital to find out what has been taken and how much, so that severity, treatment, and possible complications can be accurately assessed. Look around and gather evidence such as pill bottles, containers, and prescriptions.

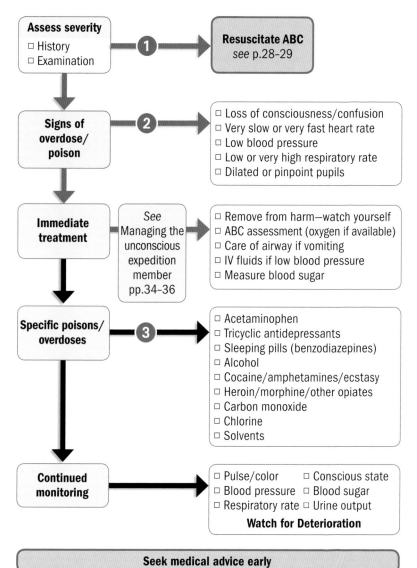

Assess severity		Resuscitate ABC
□ History □ Examination	**1**	see p.28–29

Signs of overdose/ poison — **2**
- □ Loss of consciousness/confusion
- □ Very slow or very fast heart rate
- □ Low blood pressure
- □ Low or very high respiratory rate
- □ Dilated or pinpoint pupils

Immediate treatment
See Managing the unconscious expedition member pp.34–36
- □ Remove from harm—watch yourself
- □ ABC assessment (oxygen if available)
- □ Care of airway if vomiting
- □ IV fluids if low blood pressure
- □ Measure blood sugar

Specific poisons/ overdoses — **3**
- □ Acetaminophen
- □ Tricyclic antidepressants
- □ Sleeping pills (benzodiazepines)
- □ Alcohol
- □ Cocaine/amphetamines/ecstasy
- □ Heroin/morphine/other opiates
- □ Carbon monoxide
- □ Chlorine
- □ Solvents

Continued monitoring
- □ Pulse/color   □ Conscious state
- □ Blood pressure   □ Blood sugar
- □ Respiratory rate □ Urine output

Watch for Deterioration

Seek medical advice early

1 History and examination

□ Make sure you do not become poisoned yourself.
□ If everyone is ill, consider carbon monoxide/chlorine fumes.
□ Look around for empty pill bottles/packets/prescriptions/syringes/needles.

Important points in the history	Important points in the examination
□ The casualty may be able to tell you everything □ Ask about previous medical problems □ Normal medications—check whether any are "slow-release" forms The casualty may get worse □ Alcohol is often taken with a deliberate overdose	**Look** □ Conscious state (confusion) □ Very pink or pale □ Pupils—large or small/reactive **Feel** □ Peripheral perfusion □ Brisk reflexes, tremor **Document** Blood sugar, consciousness

2 Signs of overdose

Opiates (morphine/heroin) Loss of consciousness (LoC), low blood pressure (BP), low respiratory rate, very small pupils

Tricyclic antidepressants LoC, fast heart rate, large pupils, brisk reflexes

Sleeping pills (benzodiazepine), alcohol, tricyclic antidepressants (severe): LoC, low BP, low respiratory rate, smallish pupils, floppy

Cocaine, amphetamines Agitation, tremor, sweating, fast hr, nausea, fever, big pupils

Carbon monoxide poisoning LoC, low BP, fast respiratory rate, stiff muscles, brisk reflexes, pale or flushed (cherry red)

3 Specific poisons/overdoses

If there are symptoms of overdose, seek medical advice and evacuate urgently.

Acetaminophen
Acetaminophen has no initial effect (casualty appears normal), but poisons the liver (sometimes fatally) over several days. Seek urgent medical advice.

Tricyclic antidepressants
These drugs come in many different forms but have similar effects in overdose.

Symptoms and signs	Treatment
□ LoC, confusion, large pupils, fever □ Fast heart rate but low BP with large overdose	□ Supportive—keep airway clear and ensure vomit is not inhaled. □ May need IV fluid if low BP

Sleeping pills (benzodiazepines—temazepam, diazepam, nitrazepam)
Benzodiazepines in overdose will anesthetize the casualty.

Symptoms and signs	Treatment
□ Sleepy, then LoC □ Low BP and respiratory rate □ Smallish pupils, floppy body	□ Supportive—keep airway clear and ensure vomit isn't inhaled □ Flumazenil is an antidote, but seek medical advice first

Alcohol

Overdose of alcohol (usually spirits) is common. Pills are often taken at the same time.

Symptoms and signs	Treatment
□ Sleepy then LoC, smallish pupils	□ Supportive—keep airway clear
□ Low BP, respiratory rate, blood sugar	□ May need IV fluid if BP is low
□ Look for other poisoning/smell	□ May need sugar (not oral in LoC)

Cocaine/amphetamines/ecstasy

Major overdoses may result in LoC, which is grave.

Symptoms and signs	Treatment
□ Agitation, tremor, sweating, heat	□ Keep cool—tepid cloths, fan
□ Fast pulse, dilated pupils	□ IV access and fluids
□ Seizures in severe overdose	□ Seek medical advice

Opiates (morphine, heroin)

Opiates may be taken by mouth, smoked, or injected.

Symptoms and signs	Treatment
□ Pinpoint pupils, sleepy, then LoC	□ Supportive—keep airway clear
□ Low BP and respiratory rate	□ Naloxone is an antidote, but only
□ Look for injection marks, needles	give under medical supervision

Carbon monoxide poisoning

Poisoning by carbon monoxide has an insidious onset—entire team may be affected.

Symptoms and signs	Treatment
□ Lethargy, headache, vomiting	□ Watch yourself
□ Fast respiratory rate, chest pain	□ Get casualty out of danger, give
□ Low BP and LoC, possible seizures	oxygen
□ Pale or (more serious) flushed	□ Supportive—clear airway
□ Outlook is grave in LoC	□ Treat seizures (see p.38)

Chlorine

Leaking battery acid can cause chlorine poisoning—sealed batteries are safer.

Symptoms and signs	Treatment
□ Wheeze, cough, breathlessness	□ Watch yourself
□ Chest pain	□ Get casualty out of danger and
□ Watering, sore eyes	give oxygen
□ Breathlessness may worsen over	□ Albuterol inhaler 2 puffs/15 mins
several hours	□ Prednisolone 60mg orally
	□ Evacuate before casualty worsens

Solvents (methanol, ethylene glycol)

Solvents may cause deliberate or accidental overdose. Label containers clearly.

Symptoms and signs	Treatment
□ Nausea, vomiting, low BP	□ Supportive—keep airway clear
□ Confusion, possible seizures, LoC	□ Check blood sugar (see p.50)
□ Low or high blood sugar	□ If methanol or ethylene glycol
□ Effects may be delayed up to	poisoning, give 150ml gin/
36 hours	vodka/ whisky (only if conscious)

PSYCHOLOGICAL DISORDERS

Facing the challenge of an expedition, team members will usually demonstrate their best qualities, but in rare cases may demonstrate their worst. If you gather the team together beforehand, it will help you to identify any potential conflict and take note of any members who may need extra help and advice.

Prevention

The physical and emotional strain of expeditions may heighten existing tensions. If there are major disagreements or conflicts before departing, one option is to change members, but this is a drastic measure. Find out if any team members have been treated for conditions such as depression or anxiety attacks in the past. Prevention strategies include:

□ Recognizing tiredness; ensuring as far as possible that all members of the team are sleeping, eating and drinking properly
□ Acknowledging that there are likely to be hitches and setbacks during the expedition and that plans sometimes change
□ Being vigilant against isolation or withdrawal
□ Assigning tasks and roles appropriate to each person's capabilities
□ Keeping a sense of perspective and a sense of humor.

Depression

Outward signs of depression include isolation, withdrawal, poor appetite, poor sleep, lethargy and tearfulness. The member may have been treated for similar episodes in the past. Find out whether the member has been prescribed medication for depression. If so, check that he or she is taking the correct dose. Take steps to prevent the member from being isolated; in particular, they should have a friend they can confide in. A particular trigger may have precipitated the symptoms. Investigate any solutions to existing problems.

Anxiety and panic attacks

In a challenging or unfamiliar environment, setbacks such as extreme weather and accidents are likely to cause stress. A person with acute anxiety will experience exaggerated feelings of dread, tearfulness and feelings of helplessness. Physical symptoms include fast heart rate, breathlessness and dizziness. If these symptoms are recognized, put the expedition member in a safe place until the crisis is over (for example, a quiet tent), and reassure them. In emergencies, diazepam (5mg orally as needed) can be used to control the symptoms.

Sleep disorders

Long flights, changes of time zone, hard work and disturbed sleep may all combine to cause fatigue, which quickly affects morale and decreases performance. It is important to avoid falling into a pattern of poor sleep, so make an effort to begin the expedition well rested. It is a good idea to establish a rota for cooking, washing and collecting fuel to ensure that everyone contributes and everyone gets enough rest. Sleep disorders are common at altitude—see p.59.

RESUSCITATION PROCEDURES

Basic resuscitation skills are relatively easy to learn and will improve the chances of survival should a casualty collapse. The first steps are to protect the spine, establish a clear airway and check breathing.

Once you are properly trained, it is vitally important to practice resuscitation skills often, so that you can be effective when faced with an unconscious casualty.

Control and stabilization of the cervical spine (neck)

- ☐ In trauma situations, there may be injury to the cervical spine that is not obvious.
- ☐ Avoid any unnecessary movement of the head and cervical spine and immobilize (as outlined below) as soon as possible. If you need to move the casualty away from danger, some maneuvering may be unavoidable, but try to keep it to a minimum.
- ☐ Manual immobilization of the cervical spine is only the first step. Full immobilization involves fitting a semi-rigid collar around the neck and strapping the casualty to a spinal board (*see* pp.178–79).

Immobilizing the cervical spine with your hands
- ☐ Hold firmly but gently. If the casualty is conscious, reassure them by explaining what you are doing.
- ☐ Do not let go. You are responsible for the position of the cervical spine.
- ☐ Do not cover the ears with your hands. This may cause feelings of claustrophobia.

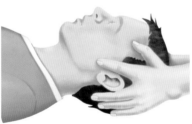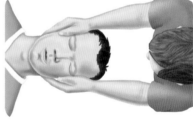

Hold the head without covering the ears, to avoid causing feelings of claustrophobia.

Position yourself comfortably and keep the head as still as possible.

Opening the airway and checking for breathing

There are two basic maneuvers you can try. Start with the combined head tilt and chin lift. Assess whether you have been successful at opening the airway and whether or not the casualty is breathing.
- ☐ Look at the chest for movement.
- ☐ Listen with your ear next to the mouth for breath sounds.
- ☐ Feel with your cheek next to the mouth for movement of air.
If there are no signs of breathing, try the jaw thrust (*see* opposite page), and reassess the breathing.

Head tilt and chin lift

☐ Place two fingers under the chin and pull the chin up.

☐ Put your hand on the forehead and push backward so the head is tilted as in the diagram.

☐ If you can, perform these maneuvers with a pillow or similar padding under the head.

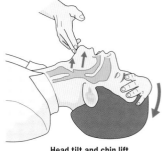
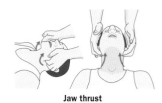

Head tilt and chin lift

Jaw thrust

☐ Put two fingers behind the "corner" of the jaw, under the ear, on each side.

☐ Push the jaw forward, so the lower teeth sit in front of the upper teeth.

☐ Reassess for breathing.

Jaw thrust

Using equipment to keep the airway open

Oropharyngeal and nasopharyngeal airway devices are simple to insert and will help to keep the air passage open. When the casualty is breathing without your help, your hands will be available for other tasks.

Inserting a oropharyngeal (Guedel) airway

☐ Do not push the tongue back in the mouth.

☐ Do not insert in a semiconscious casualty—they may vomit.

☐ In general use a size 3 (usually green) for women and a size 4 (usually orange) for men.

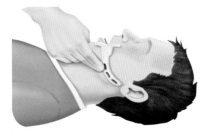

Size the airway—length should match the distance from corner of mouth to ear lobe.

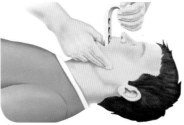

Insert the airway upside down. Do not force.

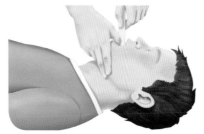

Gradually rotate the device into the correct position as you insert it.

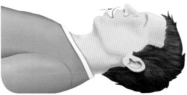

The flange should sit against the front teeth once the airway is correctly in place.

Inserting a nasopharyngeal (NP) airway

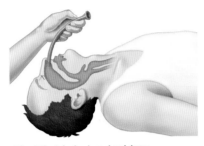

Direct the tube backward and down.

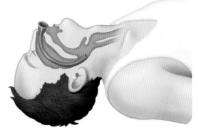

When the airway is in, only the flange will show.

- ☐ Measure a length of the NP airway equal to the distance from the side of the nose to the ear lobe. Try a size 5 for women and a size 6 for men.
- ☐ Put lubricant on the airway.
- ☐ Insert the airway toward the back of the head, not the top. Do not force.
- ☐ When the airway is position, the flange should sit at the nostril opening.
- ☐ If a safety pin comes with the airway, insert it into the flange before you put the airway in, to prevent it from disappearing up the nose.

Note Never use an NP airway if you suspect the casualty may have a basal skull fracture. Signs of basal skull fracture include obvious injury to the face, bruising around the eyes, bruising behind the ears and clear fluid coming from the nose.

How to give rescue breaths

- ☐ Establish an airway and check for breathing (see pp.172–73).
- ☐ Use a pocket mask when giving mouth-to-mouth if possible (see below left), to prevent infection. If available, administer oxygen through a tube positioned under the side of the mask.
- ☐ You can perform rescue breaths from a position beside the casualty or above the head. Keep the airway open by maintaining head tilt, chin lift or jaw thrust.

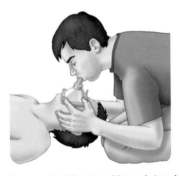

If your medical kit comes with a pocket mask, using this will help to prevent infections.

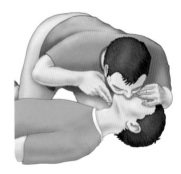

Make sure the airway remains open, maintaining a head tilt and chin lift if necessary.

- ☐ Using steady but gentle breaths, blow into the mask or mouth for 1–2 seconds and watch the casualty's chest to see it rising. Hold the nose firmly while you blow, to prevent the air from escaping.
- ☐ The chest should rise an inch or so. When it does, stop blowing and watch it fall.
- ☐ If you have to blow very hard and the chest does not rise and fall easily, the airway is not open. Adjust the head position to open the airway.

How to give a chest thump

□ Only give a chest thump if you have witnessed the collapse, the casualty is unresponsive and there is no breathing/pulse.

□ Lie the casualty facing upward on a firm surface, protecting the cervical spine if appropriate.

□ Thump the center of the chest once, firmly, with your closed fist.

□ Check for breathing and pulse. If there is no response, continue with basic and advanced life support (*see* pp.28-29).

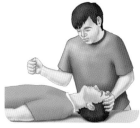

Use your closed fist to give a firm thump to the center of the chest.

How to give chest compressions

□ Lie the casualty facing upward on a firm surface, protecting the cervical spine if appropriate.

□ Assess breathing and pulse (*see* pp.180-81).

□ Clasp your hands with the heel of the lower hand on the center of the chest between the nipples (*see* illustration, right).

□ With straight arms, push down on the chest, aiming to depress the center of the chest by 2 inches (less for smaller adults). Repeat at a rate of 100 times per minute.

□ After 30 compressions, give 2 rescue breaths. Continue chest compressions with a ratio of 30 compressions to 2 rescue breaths.

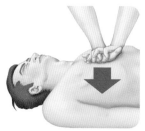

Apply pressure with the heel of one hand.

Safe defibrillation

□ Lie the casualty facing upward on a firm surface, protecting the cervical spine if appropriate.

□ Assess breathing and pulse (*see* pp.180-81). Continue chest compressions until the AED is attached to the casualty.

□ Make sure the casualty is dry, the surface the casualty is lying on is dry and you are dry.

□ Attach one defibrillator pad just below the collar bone on the right side of the chest and the other below and to the side of the left nipple (not on the breast in women)—*see* illustration, below right.

□ Remove the oxygen mask and put it somewhere out of the way.

□ Switch on the AED (refer to the manual that accompanies the AED beforehand).

□ **MAKE SURE EVERYONE IS WELL AWAY FROM THE CASUALTY BEFORE DEFIBRILLATING TO AVOID RISK OF ACCIDENTAL SHOCK**

□ After defibrillation, immediately continue with life support—follow the AED instructions.

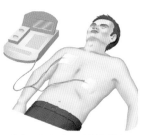

Automated external defibrillator

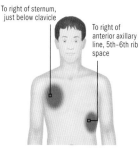

To right of sternum, just below clavicle

To right of anterior axillary line, 5th-6th rib space

Sites for defibrillator pads

RECOVERY POSITION AND LOG ROLL

Recovery position

A casualty who is unconscious or semiconscious as a result of accident or illness may not be able to maintain their own airway. The following problems may occur:
□ The tongue may fall back and block the airway
□ Saliva may trickle down into the trachea (wind pipe) and lungs
□ Refluxing stomach acid and vomit may also pass into the lungs.
If the lungs become contaminated with secretions or vomit, this will cause a chest infection and threaten recovery. Stomach acid can reflux into the mouth and from there enter the lungs without any outward sign, particularly if the casualty is unconscious.

Method

□ Ensure the casualty is stable, has an open airway, is breathing and has a pulse.
□ Leave any airway devices in place (see pp.173–74).
□ Use the log roll (see opposite page) if the casualty may have sustained a spinal injury.
□ Straighten the casualty's arms and legs, making sure the spine is protected. Move the arm nearest to you up, so that the hand is beside the head (**1**).

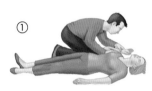

□ Bring the opposite arm across the casualty's body, and place the back of the hand against the cheek on your side.
□ Bend the opposite leg up at the knee (**2**). With one hand on the bent knee, use the leg as a lever, to rotate the casualty toward you gently; place the other hand on the far shoulder and bring the upper body toward you at the same time (**3**). Control the rotation with your knees.

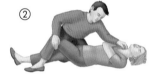

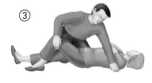

□ Place the head comfortably on the back of one hand, and position the bent upper leg far enough forward to prevent the body from rolling in either direction (**4**).

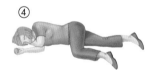

□ The arms and upper leg should form right angles, to provide the best support.

Notes

□ Assess for ABC frequently (see p.28–29).
□ The recovery position is quite stable, and the casualty can stay in this position for a few hours. For extra security place rolled-up sleeping bags or something similar on either side of the casualty.
□ Injured limbs may require additional support—use something firm but not hard.
□ Move the casualty every two to three hours to relieve pressure points.

Modified recovery position
Extend the arm closest to you straight above the casualty's head. Log roll the casualty toward you onto their side, and rest the head on the extended arm. Either keep the legs straight or bend them to improve stability. Use sleeping bags, bedding or anything similar you have to hand to support the casualty in position. Turn the casualty every few hours to prevent pressure sores from developing.

Log roll

Always use a log roll to turn a casualty if you suspect a spinal injury. You might also use a log roll for the following reasons:
☐ To examine the back of the casualty for injuries
☐ To place the casualty in a modified recovery position while waiting to evacuate
☐ To position a recovery stretcher underneath the casualty.
A log roll should be performed by at least three people. If you only have two, perform the roll as best you can (see illustration below). Having four people is ideal, so that three can roll and the fourth can examine. The objective of the log roll is to keep the entire spine in one line (not just the neck). Fit a semi-rigid collar to the neck before rolling if possible, to protect the cervical spine (see p.178).

Method
☐ Position yourselves as illustrated below, kneeling and stable.
☐ The first person guides the roll and immobilizes the cervical spine, with or without a semi-rigid collar. This person controls all movements and must be very clear in giving instructions to the others.
☐ The second person places one hand on the casualty's shoulder and one hand on the top of the thigh.
☐ The third person puts one hand on the top of the pelvis, above the lower hand of the second person, and the other hand on the lower leg, just below the knee.
☐ On the command of the first person, smoothly rotate the casualty by 90°, so that they come to rest against the knees of person two and person three.
☐ Hold the casualty in position until the examination is complete or the spinal board or stretcher is in place beneath them.
☐ When the first person gives the command, smoothly rotate the casualty back into the original position, lying on their back.

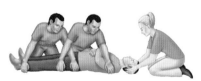 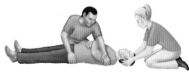

Log roll technique with three people: one person stabilizes the neck.

Log roll technique with two people: a third may examine the back.

Notes
☐ It is important to be able to see the casualty's face at all times, so that you can assess for breathing, vomit and secretions.
☐ If only three people can help, two may need to log roll while the third examines.

SPINAL IMMOBILIZATION

Full immobilization of the spine involves fitting a semi-rigid collar to the neck, strapping the casualty to a long spinal board, and securing the head with side blocks and straps/tape.

Indications for immobilizing the spine

- ☐ Obvious head or neck trauma
- ☐ Injury to the upper chest
- ☐ Injury to another part of the spine
- ☐ Numbness or tingling in the limbs after an accident

- ☐ An accident of strong impact, such as a fall from a height >3m or a collision with a vehicle
- ☐ Trauma involving multiple injuries
- ☐ Injury to the pelvis

> **If in doubt, immobilize the casualty with a semi-rigid collar and spinal board.**

Fitting a semi-rigid collar

Maintain manual immobilization of the cervical spine while the collar is being fitted; continue supporting the neck until the casualty is fully immobilized on a spinal board or similar long board—*see* opposite.

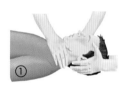

Method
- ☐ Measure the distance between the jaw line and the top of shoulders in finger widths (**1**). Match this height with the hard plastic part of the collar that fits over the shoulder, beneath the ear. Collars come in various fixed sizes or may be adjustable—follow sizing instructions.
- ☐ Slide the back of the collar under the neck all the way through to the other side (**2**).
- ☐ Rotate the front part over the neck, ensuring that the chin rest fits snugly under the chin, lifting it somewhat, so that the head is tilted back slightly (**3**).
- ☐ Secure the back of the collar using the hook-and-loop tape attached for this purpose.
- ☐ Ask the casualty if the collar feels comfortable—secure but not too tight. If the casualty is unconscious, try to insert your finger between the casualty's skin and the collar; it should fit without you having to force it.
- ☐ Complete immobilization by securing the casualty to a spinal board (**4**).

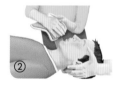

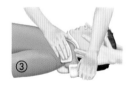

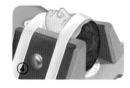

Notes
- ☐ Semi-rigid collars can cause pressure sores if left on for too long. Loosen the collar for a few minutes every two hours until the casualty is evacuated.
- ☐ A tightly rolled towel can be used in place of a cervical collar. Wrap the towel around the neck, under the chin, and tape it in position.

Immobilizing a casualty on a spinal board

- The first step is to immobilize the cervical spine, using either a purpose-designed semi-rigid collar or an improvised collar, such as a rolled towel.
- After stabilizing the cervical spine, the second step is ABCDE assessment (see p.29–33). This takes priority over placing the casualty on a spinal board.
- When these actions are completed, move the casualty onto the spinal board as soon as possible. Keep the casualty in this position for a maximum of 2 hours only, to prevent pressure sores from developing.

Method

- Log roll the casualty onto one side (see p.177).
- Position the spinal board securely under the casualty as far as it will go, without moving the casualty.
- Smoothly rotate the casualty until they are facing upward on the board.
- If you need to slide the casualty further onto the board, keep the cervical spine immobilized and, on command, gently slide the casualty fully onto the board, keeping the entire spine in line.

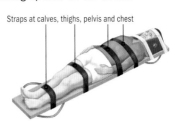

Straps at calves, thighs, pelvis and chest

Full spinal immobilization

- Keeping the cervical spine immobilized, secure straps in these positions:
  - Around the upper chest, including the arms
  - Around the pelvis, including the arms
  - Around the thighs
  - Around the calves
- Make sure the straps are secure but not too tight, so they don't restrict breathing.
- Fix padded blocks or rolled towels on either side of the head.
- Secure straps over the forehead and over the front part of the collar.
- When this process is completed, manual immobilization can be released. The casualty is ready to be transported on the board.

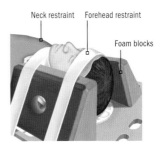

Neck restraint   Forehead restraint

Foam blocks

Immobilizing the head and neck on a spinal board

Notes

- Be very cautious about vomiting, because the casualty cannot move. Turn the board on its side immediately to prevent vomit from entering the lungs.
- Being immobilized may cause feelings of claustrophobia and the casualty may struggle, especially if disorientated. Small amounts of diazepam may be needed (2mg intravenously every 30 minutes as needed), but seek medical advice first. Be very careful about sedating brain-injured casualties.
- A spinal board can be improvised from any long board. Use duct tape or another suitable method to strap the casualty in position. Place a foam mat or sleeping bag under the casualty to ease pressure points.
- The casualty should only remain on a spinal board for a maximum of 2 hours before being transfered to a firm mattress on level ground.

PULSE AND BLOOD PRESSURE

Pulse and blood pressure are basic vital signs, giving an important indication of the functioning of the heart, or, more accurately, the cardiovacular system. Knowing how to measure these signs correctly is essential.

General appearance If a casualty is unwell, they will often have a pale appearance and cold hands and feet. A casualty who has suffered a cardiac arrest will look white.

Pulse An unwell casualty may have a very slow pulse rate (<45 beats per minute) or a very fast pulse rate (>130 beats per minute).

Blood pressure In a casualty who is injured or unwell, the blood pressure may be low (<90mmHg systolic pressure) or very high (>160mmHg systolic pressure).

Perfusion of the skin Blood flow to the skin may be reduced, particularly if a casualty is in shock (capillary refill time >4 seconds–see opposite page).

Measuring the pulse

- □ The pulse can be checked in any area of the the body where an artery lies close to the skin.
- □ Feel for the pulse firmly with two fingers, but do not press too hard or you may restrict the blood supply to that area.
- □ Count for 30 seconds, using a watch or a clock with a second hand.
- □ Be accurate. If you estimate, you may draw false conclusions and adversely affect treatment.

IN AN EMERGENCY

Measure the carotid pulse
Feel for the pulse in the groove between the larynx (voice box) and the muscles of the neck.

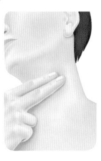

Measure the femoral pulse
Feel for the pulse in the skin groove in the groin, at the top of the leg.

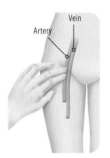

IN A ROUTINE CHECK

Measure the radial pulse
Feel for the pulse at the wrist, in the groove about 3cm proximal from the base of the thumb.

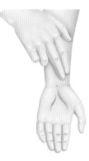

Measure the brachial pulse
Feel for the pulse at the elbow, on the inside edge of the bicep.

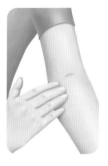

Measuring blood pressure

The blood pressure has two values. In the example 120/70mmHg:
Systolic blood pressure (SBP)—is the higher value (120mmHg).
Diastolic blood pressure (DBP)—is the lower value (70mmHg).

Method
- [ ] Position the casualty sitting down or lying down if necessary.
- [ ] Fasten the cuff snugly around the upper arm. Larger people need larger cuffs.
- [ ] Make sure you can feel a clear radial pulse, then begin to pump the cuff, continuing to feel for the pulse.
- [ ] Note the pressure on the dial (in mmHg) when you lose the pulse. Inflate the cuff a further 20–30mmHg and then very slowly, still feeling the pulse, release the air from the cuff with the screw valve.
- [ ] The pressure at which the pulse reappears is the SBP.
- [ ] Inflate the cuff to 20–30mmHg above the SBP, and listen with a stethoscope over the brachial artery. Let the air out slowly.
- [ ] At about the SBP, you will hear a tapping noise made by the pulse reappearing in the brachial artery.
- [ ] Continue to release the air slowly, listening to the tapping noise. When the tapping stops note the pressure. This is the DBP.

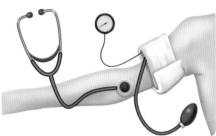

Inflatable cuff and bulb, stethoscope and measurement dial

Estimating the blood pressure

If it is not possible to measure the blood pressure using the technique above, you can estimate the SBP by checking various pulses (*see* opposite for locations):
If a radial pulse is present: SBP >70mmHg
If a brachial pulse is present: SBP >60mmHg
If a carotid pulse is present: SBP >50mmHg
Remember, these are only estimates. Assess the person as a whole.

Automated blood pressure measurement

Many medical kits contain an automated device for measuring blood pressure. Most of these devices are easy to operate, but instructions should accompany the device. If the blood pressure is very low or if the pulse is irregular, it may be more difficult to take a reading.

Capillary refill time (CRT)

Measuring the capillary refill time is a way of assessing the supply of blood to the skin, which is useful for checking general blood supply and indicating the degree of shock. Capillary refill may naturally take longer if the casualty is very cold.
- [ ] Press on the end of a finger (the fleshy part) or the forehead for 4 seconds.
- [ ] Release and time how long it takes for the white "blanch" mark to pink up again.
- [ ] Refill should take less than 2 seconds. If the CRT is longer than 4 seconds, the casualty may require IV fluids (*see* p.186).

ASSESSING CONSCIOUS STATE: GLASGOW COMA SCALE (GCS) AND AVPU

Monitoring the conscious state of a sick or injured team member will allow you to detect improvement or deterioration and report accurately to medical authorities. The possible levels of consciousness range from being completely awake and alert to being deeply unconscious and unrousable.

AVPU and the GCS are methods of assessing the conscious state and giving it a value. Repeating the measurement over time allows you to detect deterioration or improvement and take appropriate action. AVPU is a quick, straightforward system for scoring the conscious state. GCS is a more comprehensive and sensitive method but requires more skill and time. Small changes in conscious state are more likely to be detected by calculating GCS.

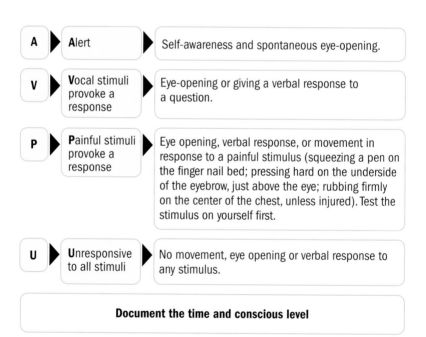

A	**A**lert	Self-awareness and spontaneous eye-opening.
V	**V**ocal stimuli provoke a response	Eye-opening or giving a verbal response to a question.
P	**P**ainful stimuli provoke a response	Eye opening, verbal response, or movement in response to a painful stimulus (squeezing a pen on the finger nail bed; pressing hard on the underside of the eyebrow, just above the eye; rubbing firmly on the center of the chest, unless injured). Test the stimulus on yourself first.
U	**U**nresponsive to all stimuli	No movement, eye opening or verbal response to any stimulus.

Document the time and conscious level

Glasgow Coma Scale

☐ GCS scores the eye, motor and verbal responses to stimulation and combines the results for an overall measure of concious state.
☐ The response that should be recorded is the best one the casualty gives. For example, if the casualty has one injured arm and one uninjured arm, you would score the response of the uninjured arm.
☐ Obeying a command might include poking the tongue out or opening or closing the eyes on request.
☐ If the casualty speaks clearly in a foreign language, score them normally, regardless of whether you understand the words.

	Best Response	Score
Eyes	Eyes open spontaneously	4
	Eyes open on being asked a question	3
	Eyes open on painful stimulus	2
	Eyes stay shut	1
Motor	Obeys commands (squeezes hands, pokes tongue out)	6
	Moves hand to stop painful stimulus (localizes)	5
	Withdraws hand/arm or leg from painful stimulus	4
	Bends up arms and legs to painful stimulus	3
	Straightens arms and legs to painful stimulus	2
	No movement of any part of the body to any stimulus	1
Verbal	Gives answers to questions, seems oriented	5
	Answers questions but shows confusion	4
	Speaks in single words, no sentences	3
	Makes incomprehensible sounds	2
	Gives no verbal response	1
The maximum GCS is 15	Fully awake and not confused	
The minimum GCS is 3	Deeply unconscious and unresponsive	

Notes
☐ A GCS of 8 or less suggests that the casualty is unconscious. In this state, they may not be able to maintain a clear airway independently. They may inhale vomit or secretions into the lungs, or the tongue may fall back and obstruct the airway. Place the casualty in the recovery position (see pp.176-77).
☐ Check that injuries are not intefering with the assessment: paralyzed limbs, facial swelling and mouth injuries can all prevent the casualty from giving a response that accurately reflects their conscious level.
☐ A change of 2 or more in the GCS implies a significant change in conscious level.

Document the time and the total score.
Also note the scores for each separate response

REHYDRATION

Injury and illness can hinder the body's ability to maintain an appropriate level of hydration. In a hospital, sterile fluid can usually be infused directly into a casualty's blood vessels through a cannula inserted into a vein. In the wilderness, however, you may not have the equipment and expertise necessary for administering IV fluids.

Other options for rehydrating a casualty include the oral route, a nasogastric tube and, if other methods are not possible, the rectal route. The same types of fluid can be used for these three alternative methods.

Oral route Giving fluids by mouth is the most effective and convenient way of rehydrating a casualty. The fluid should be clean, but does not have to be sterile. If severe diarrhea, vomiting and/or sweating occurs, DO NOT USE WATER ALONE. Administer a solution that will replace lost chemicals (see opposite page). If the casualty is not fully conscious, DO NOT USE THE ORAL ROUTE—vomit may enter the lungs. If the casualty is awake and vomiting only occasionally, persist with oral fluids at first. Give the casualty antinausea drugs to prevent vomiting.

Nasogastric (NG) tube (see p.200) An NG tube can be used in an unconscious casualty but not if they are vomiting, so administer antinausea medication (see pp.226–30). A disadvangate of NG tubes is that they can be difficult to insert.

Rectal route (see p.202) The rectal route is the next option to try if intractable vomiting occurs or if IV access is impossible. This method can be effective, but less fluid is likely to be absorbed than by the oral or NG route.

Routine fluid loss per day for a typical 70kg person

Route of loss	Amount lost per day (ml)
Perspiration (no work)	700
Breath	500
Urine	1300
Feces	100
TOTAL	**2600ml/day**

Note Losses caused by perspiration (particularly in hot climates and with physical exertion) may increase to above 5000ml.

Daily fluid requirements

For the average-sized man: 3000ml/day
For the average-sized woman: 2200ml/day
These amounts fulfil the body's normal daily requirements (see opposite for guidance on giving extra fluid).

Reasons for emergency rehydration

- Severe vomiting
- Profuse diarrhea
- Blood loss
- Severe heat illness
- Burns
- Diabetic crisis
- Hydration for unconscious casualty
- Shock (other causes)

Emergency rehydration

Circumstances will dictate the amount of fluid required.

Immediately Give 500ml of fluid by the simplest route available (IV if unconscious).

Assess Check the casualty's level of hydration/shock (*see* below).

Check medical history If the casualty has heart, lung or kidney disease, seek medical advice before administering more than 1L of fluid.

Continue giving fluid until signs of shock reduce If the casualty is still exhibiting signs of shock after being given 1.5L of fluid, seek medical advice.

Maintain daily requirements Give fluids until casualty is drinking well or evacuated.

Estimating and replacing blood loss

- Estimating blood loss is difficult. Estimate in 250ml amounts (approximately one cup)—for example, blood loss may be estimated at 250ml, 500ml or 750ml.
- For every **1000ml blood loss**, the casualty requires **3000ml fluid replacement** with a clear crystalloid solution (such as Ringer's Lactate or 0.9% saline solution).
- If you use colloid solutions (for example, gelatin, dextran or starch solutions) give 1000ml solution per 1000ml of blood loss initially and then reassess. The casualty will probably need more.

Assessing level of hydration

Signs of continued dehydration include:
- Fast pulse rate (>100bpm)
- Low blood pressure
- Pale/white skin
- Cold skin on distal arms and legs
- Dark urine (should be pale or colorless)
- Urine output less than 30ml/hour for average-sized adult.

Emergency mixture for oral/NG/rectal fluid rehydration

Use premade oral rehydration salts (ORS) such as those produced by the World Health Organization. Alternate 1L ORS and then 1L water.

OR

Emergency ORS solution:
- 1L clean water
- Add 6–8 level teaspoons of sugar (or 2 teaspoons of honey)
- Add 1–2 level teaspoons of table salt
- Add a generous squeeze of lemon/orange/lime/grapefruit juice or a spoonful of mashed banana
- Taste the mixture yourself first: it should be slightly salty.

VENOUS AND INTRAOSSEOUS ACCESS

IV route

The venous route is very effective for delivering fluids or drugs directly into the circulation, and they can begin to work within minutes. Inserting a cannula requires training, however, and once learned, the skills should be practiced regularly. There are risks involved in using a cannula (see opposite), so observe good hygiene and wear gloves.

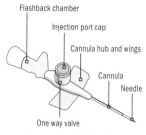

Flashback chamber

Injection port cap

Cannula hub and wings

Cannula

Needle

One way valve

Cannula for IV fluid and drugs

Inserting a cannula

Method

☐ Fix a tourniquet firmly around the upper arm (**1**). If necessary, someone can put their hands around the arm to act as a tourniquet.

☐ Wait for a few minutes for the veins to appear.
- Ask the casualty to clench and unclench their hand to bring the veins up.
- Tap the veins, which will make them expand.
- Hang the arm down so blood runs into the arm.

☐ Clean the skin over a suitable vein with an antiseptic swab or solution. Wear sterile gloves.

☐ Gently stretch the skin on either side of the vein and pull it toward you (**2**). Do not touch the cannula, only the hub.

☐ Line the cannula up with the vein, at an angle of about 30° to the skin.

☐ Insert the tip of the cannula through the skin, and then reduce the angle to about 15° (**3**).

☐ Advance slowly into the vein. Watch the back end of the cannula very carefully. When you see a flash of blood, stop advancing immediately.

☐ Hold the back end of the needle very still and advance the wings or hub of the cannula so the plastic tube goes into the vein (**4**). The tube should advance easily. If it does not, start again.

☐ Release the tourniquet.

☐ Take the stopper off the back end of the needle and screw it to the end of the cannula.

☐ Fix the cannula in place securely with a cannula-fixing dressing or with purpose-designed tape (**5**).

☐ Flush the cannula with a 5ml syringe of saline. The saline should go in easily and should not cause swelling or pain.

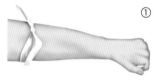

①

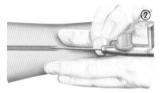

②

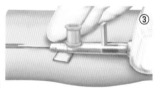

③

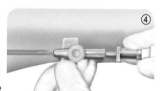

④

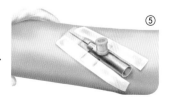

⑤

Cautions and complications
- Larger cannulas deliver a higher volume of fluid but are more difficult to put in.
- Only give sterile fluid that is intended for IV use.
- Beware: no air should enter the cannula, as it may cause cardiac arrest or stroke.
- Watch for signs of infection including red skin, pain on injection, swelling and blockage. If any of these signs occur, remove the cannula.
- The cannula can remain in place for 5 days, unless it becomes infected, painful or blocked. If it does, remove it earlier and insert a new one in a different place.

Sites for inserting a cannula
- Back of hand: good for normal IV fluids and drugs
- Wrist: suitable for resuscitating fluids and larger cannulas
- Inside of the elbow: veins are larger, so it is easier to insert the canula, but the arm must stay straight
- Feet/lower leg: these sites can also be considered.

Intraosseous (IO) access

Consider IO access in emergency situations if IV access is not possible. This technique allows fast fluid replacement through an IO needle (1L every 30 minutes) and administration of epinephrine and atropine. Gaining access involves inserting a needle directly into the bone—usually just below the knee on the inside of the tibia (shin bone). Once in place, the IO needle can be used for several hours before being replaced with IV access. IO access requires a special hollow needle with a trocar. There are also specialized devices that "fire" the needle into the bone. DO NOT USE if the leg has a suspected fracture, infected skin, an open wound, infected bone or known osteoporosis.

Method for gaining IO access
- Wear sterile gloves and clean the skin first with an antiseptic cleansing solution.
- Identify the site for needle insertion: on the flat of the inner (medial) side of the shin bone, about 5cm below the knee (in an average sized adult) (**1**).
- Support the leg behind the knee, which should be slightly bent.
- Firmly insert the needle—or "fire" the device, holding it firmly (**2**)—through the skin at right angles.
- Advance the needle into the bone, twisting it, until you feel a "give"—may be subtle.
- The needle should stay upright in the bone by itself. Remove the trocar (**3**).
- Flush the needle with 5ml saline, which should go in easily.
- Connect the infusion line to the needle and tape the line to the leg (**4**).

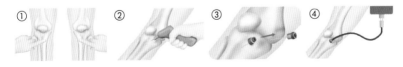

Cautions and complications
- If the leg swells around the needle or more generally, this means the needle is inserted incorrectly—stop the infusion and take it out.
- Both skin and bone can become infected, so watch for redness, swelling and pain. If these signs develop, remove the needle and treat with antibiotics.

INJECTIONS AND INFUSIONS

The three options for giving injections with a syringe and needle are: into a vein (intravenous—IV), into a muscle (intramuscular—IM) or under the skin (subcutaneous). Not all injectable drugs can be given in all three ways, so read the individual drug instructions or seek medical advice.

In an infusion, fluid is injected into a vein continually over the course of hours, or even days, through a cannula (*see* p.186 on how to insert a cannula). This process requires a particular type of tubing (known as a "giving set") and sterile fluid that is specifically designed for infusion into the vein.

General rules

□ Make sure you have the correct drug in the appropriate dosage for the casualty. Ask another team member to double check. It is easy to make a mistake.

□ Keep the procedure sterile: clean the skin beforehand with a purpose-designed alcohol wipe or a cotton swab soaked in chlorhexidine; protect the needle and syringe from contamination. Wear sterile gloves.

□ When drawing the drug up into the syringe, make sure there is no air in the barrel. To expel any air, hold the syringe needle upward and push the plunger in slowly.

□ Check the casualty afterward for signs of an allergic reaction (*see* pp.48–49).

□ Dispose of all needles and other sharp objects safely.

IV injections

The veins on the insides of the elbows are the best ones to use for IV injections, but look for other sites if you can't gain access in this area.

Syringe and needle

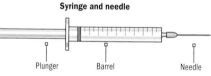

Plunger   Barrel   Needle

□ Prepare the drug and clean the skin at the injection site. Wear sterile gloves.

□ Put a tourniquet around the upper arm, and let the arm hang down to fill the veins with blood.

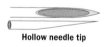

Hollow needle tip

□ Put two fingers on either side of the vein where you want to inject, and pull the skin apart and toward you.

□ Insert the needle, hole upward, at an angle of 30° to the skin (**1**), pointing up the arm (toward the heart) (**2**). Once the tip is inside the skin, pull back on the plunger slightly.

①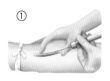

□ When the tip of the needle enters the vein, blood will appear in the syringe barrel. Stop advancing the needle. Release the tourniquet.

□ Inject the drug slowly and smoothly, checking for any swelling around the tip of the needle. Swelling indicates that the needle tip is not in the vein—start again.

②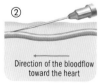

Direction of the bloodflow toward the heart

□ When you have finished injecting, remove the needle from the skin with a smooth motion, press down firmly on the injection site with a cotton swab for a few minutes then apply an adhesive bandage.

Intramuscular injections

It is easier to inject into a muscle than into a vein. DO NOT give IM if the casualty takes anticoagulants—it will bleed.

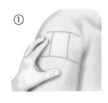

□ The two best sites for giving an IM injection are the shoulder (**1**) and the outer, upper side of the buttock (**2**) (this avoids the sciatic nerve).

□ For an adult of average size use a green (size 21 gauge) needle. For a smaller adult, use a blue (23 gauge) needle.

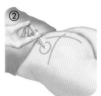

□ Clean the skin over the injection site.

□ Hold the syringe firmly by the barrel as though it were a dart, and aim it at 90° to the skin.

□ In a smooth movement, push almost the whole needle in.

□ Pull back on the plunger. If blood appears in the syringe barrel, the needle is in a blood vessel. Withdraw it 10mm, angle the needle to one side, and push it in again. Repeat until you are certain that the needle is not in a blood vessel.

□ Inject the plunger smoothly over 5 seconds (**2**).

□ Withdraw the needle and press on site with a cotton swab.

Subcutaneous injections

These are similar to IM injections but not as deep. Prepare the same way. Drug absorption may be very slow if the casualty is cold and the blood supply to the skin is limited.

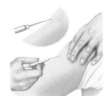

□ Use an orange (25 gauge) needle.

□ Pinch the skin on the shoulder gently between your thumb and forefinger to pull up a ridge of skin.

□ Push the needle into the skin on the top of the ridge at a low angle, to about half the length of the needle; inject smoothly over a few seconds.

Inject under the skin at a low angle.

□ Withdraw the needle and press on the site with a cotton swab.

Setting up an infusion

This is a sterile procedure so avoid touching the connectors.

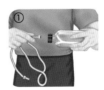

□ Find the roller valve on the giving set, and turn this off before you begin.

□ The giving set has a sharp, piercing end which should be inserted into the port on the bag or bottle of fluid (**1**).

□ Hang the bag or bottle upside down, and squeeze the lower drip chamber until it is half full of fluid (**2**).

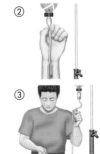

□ Open the roller valve and watch the fluid flow down the tubing to the end. Keep flushing fluid through until all the air bubbles have gone (**3**). Shut off the roller valve.

□ Connect the tubing to the cannula inserted in the vein.

□ Open the roller valve, and adjust the drip rate to deliver the desired flow rate. Tape tube to arm in two places.

□ If arm begins to swell at site of cannula, stop infusion and resite cannula.

MINOR OPERATIVE SET-UP

Wilderness surroundings and bad weather will make it more difficult to achieve a sterile environment for the occasional minor medical procedure that may be required. However, good preparation will improve the outcome

---

Procedures that might require operative set-up

☐ Wound repair (cleaning, suturing/stapling and dressing)

☐ Incising, draining and wicking an abscess

☐ Inserting a chest drain

☐ Inserting a urinary catheter

☐ Inserting a rectal rehydration tube

☐ Inserting an IV catheter

☐ Performing a nerve block

☐ Cleaning, reducing and dressing an open fracture

Preparing the casualty

☐ Explain exactly what you are going to do. Be honest about whether the procedure will be painful or not.

☐ Find a comfortable and stable position and try to put the casualty at ease: administer adequate pain relief (local anesthesia and analgesia that will be effective for a longer period); maintain privacy and dignity (avoid any flippant comments); and keep the casualty warm.

☐ Privacy and warmth are important, but you also need sufficient access to the area you will be dealing with. Expose slightly more of the body than you need to, so you won't have to make adjustments while you are wearing sterile gloves.

☐ When everything is in place, you will need to clean a good area around the site with a sterilizing skin preparation fluid. Check that the casualty is not allergic to the fluid.

Preparing yourself

☐ Ask for advice before you begin, not during or after the procedure.

☐ Ensure that you will have a comfortable and stable working position.

☐ It is probably better to have the casualty lying down rather than sitting up, in case they feel faint during the procedure.

☐ Make sure your arms are bare to above the elbow, and wash thoroughly with soap and water. If the kit contains pure alcohol or chlorhexidine, you can use one of these to sterilize your hands.

☐ When you are ready, put on a sterile pair of gloves that fit you. If there are no sterile gloves available, wear nonsterile gloves and rub your hands in sterilizing skin preparation fluid.

Preparing the set-up

□ Try to choose a well sheltered spot and wait for good weather if possible.
□ Ensure you have a trusted helper who knows what you are going to do and what you need. Don't be afraid to ask for help.
□ Set up on level ground if possible.
□ Make sure you have sufficient light—headlamps are effective.

Preparing the equipment

□ Gather all the equipment you might need before you begin.
□ Sterilize instruments by submerging them in boiling water for twenty minutes then allowing them to cool, or by washing them in sterilizing skin preparation fluid if nothing else is available. Your medical kit may include specific instrument-sterilizing fluid or sterile procedure packs, which contain a range of sterile equipment.
□ You may need:
- Sterile forceps
- Sterile scissors
- Sutures or staples and stapler
- Disposable razor (for removing hair)
- Sterile skin drape for around the site
- Sterile pot for fluid
- Sterile hemostatic clamp
- Sterile scalpel
- Sterile swabs
- Sterilizing skin preparation fluid
- Sterile drape for set-up
- Sterile tweezers
□ Use one sterile drape to make a sterile field, where you can place all equipment.
□ Make sure you choose a stable area, so the equipment doesn't fall onto the floor and get contaminated.

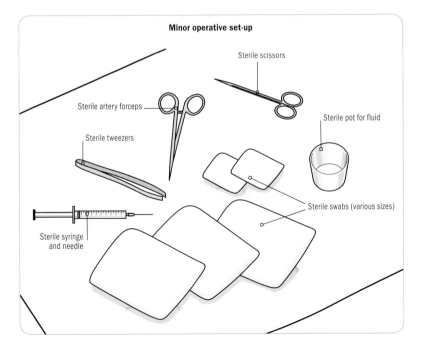

Minor operative set-up

Sterile scissors

Sterile artery forceps

Sterile pot for fluid

Sterile tweezers

Sterile swabs (various sizes)

Sterile syringe and needle

REPAIRING THE SKIN

If a deep, gaping wound is left open to heal by itself, it will leave a large scar. A wound that is neatly closed will leave only a small scar. Always use sterile gloves when repairing wounds and prepare a sterile field.

Wounds that should NOT be closed:

☐ Gaping wounds, with significant tissue loss and ragged edges
☐ Infected wounds (indicated by pus)
☐ Wounds that have been open for longer than 18 hours
☐ Wounds that are contaminated and cannot be properly cleaned, which are likely to become infected. Any sutures will need to be taken out to let pus discharge.

A wound that cannot be closed should be cleaned as thoroughly as possible and then dressed with sterile gauze and bandaging. Be gentle. Once dressed, the wound should be inspected each day and cleaned with sterile fluid. If it shows signs of infection (redness, swelling, pus), start oral antibiotics.

Methods for repairing skin wounds

Method	Difficulty	Indications	Cautions
Adhesive wound closure strips	Easy	Small incisions less than 10cm long	Not good in the damp or over joints
Skin staples	Difficult	Wounds on the trunk, scalp, arms, and legs	Do not use on face and neck
Tissue adhesive (skin glue)	Moderate	Small incisions less than 10cm in length; clean edges	Do not use in the damp or over joints; do not get in the eye
Sutures	Difficult	Large, ragged wounds; wounds in skin over joints; persistent bleeding	Use thinner thread on the face, lips (see below)

Adhesive wound closure strips

☐ Make sure bleeding has stopped and the wound is completely dry and clean.
☐ Starting at one end, use an adhesive strip to pull the edges of the wound together gently and then stick down the other side (**1**); if the edges are jagged, match the edges together and stick them in place.

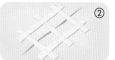

☐ Position the next strip 8-10mm from the first. If there are enough strips available, stick two strips parallel to the wound, one on either side (**2**).

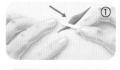

☐ Place a dressing over the wound to keep it dry and clean.
☐ Leave the strips on until they fall off. Replace the strips that fall off if the wound has not healed properly.

Skin staples

□ Position the skin edges together with the cut edges pointing to the outside, so that outer skin is not stapled inside the wound.
□ Hold the edges in place, position the stapler as shown (*see* right) and staple the skin at 7–10mm intervals.
□ If the wound has jagged edges, staple matching pieces together first, then staple from one end.
□ Place a sterile dressing over the wound.
□ Leave the staples for the same length of time as sutures (*see* below), inspecting the wound often for infection and swelling. You may need to remove staples to let pus out.

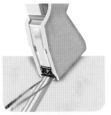

Use a pair of forceps to hold the wound edges together.

Skin glue

□ Use on straight, dry, nonbleeding cuts and not over joints.
□ Hold skin together and run glue along the wound edges.
□ Keep glue out of the cut, as it will prevent healing.
□ Apply up to three layers (read product instructions).
□ Hold the wound edges together for 30 seconds while the glue sets. Full bond should develop in 2–3 minutes.
□ A dressing is not usually needed, but keep the wound dry.
□ Adhesive should come off naturally after 7–10 days.

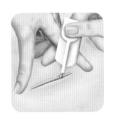

Apply skin glue on either side of the wound.

Sutures (silk, polyester or polyamide—thread bonded to a needle)

□ Use local anesthetic (up to 10ml 2% lidocaine) if putting in more than 2 sutures.
□ First, put a suture in halfway along the wound, then in each quarter, then fill in the gaps, leaving about 10mm between sutures.
□ If the wound has jagged edges, match these up first and suture them in place.
□ Use "interrupted" sutures as in (**1**): hold the skin edges up with a pair of forceps (the toothed kind work well) while you put the needle in approximately 5mm from the wound edge and curve it deeply into the skin (**2**) coming out in the middle, then put the needle through the opposite edge (**3**); aim to exit 5mm from the wound on the other side.
□ Tie with a reef knot (**4**), pulling the knot just tightly enough to bring the skin edges together and no tighter, or lack of blood flow will prevent healing.
□ If you are not satisfied with a suture, take it out and start again.
□ Clean the wound again and apply a sterile dressing.
□ Inspect every two days. If the wound looks red and swollen, release a suture and see if pus comes out. Leave the suture out and reapply a fresh dressing.

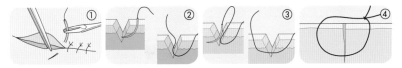

When to remove sutures and clips

□ Face: 3–5 days
□ Scalp: 7–10 days
□ Limbs: 10–14 days
□ Joints: 14 days
□ Trunk: 7–10 days

CHEST DRAINS AND DECOMPRESSION

Tension pneumothorax occurs when trapped air in the chest cavity puts pressure on the lungs and heart, eventually causing collapse and possible death (see pp.108–109). Emergency decompression may prevent collapse and needs to be followed by insertion of a chest drain if the medical kit contains the necessary equipment.

If the casualty has a suspected tension pneumothorax, after performing emergency decompression of the chest, seek medical advice immediately and arrange urgent evacuation. Blood in the chest cavity (hemothorax—see p.109) may be suspected. This condition should not require emergency decompression, but does require IV cannulation and fluids for resuscitation.

Signs of a tension pneumothorax	Signs of a hemothorax
□ Breathing difficulties □ Low blood pressure □ The trachea may be shifted away from the side of the chest with the air in it □ Reduced breath sounds on the side of the chest with the air in it	□ Breathing difficulties □ Casualty may be shocked (low blood pressure) □ Reduced breath sounds on the side of the chest with the blood in it

Emergency chest decompression

To perform decompression, insert a cannula into the front of the chest on the side where you suspect there may be a tension pneumothorax.
- □ Position the casualty in a stable position, sitting upright at a 30° angle if possible.
- □ Use sterile gloves and a sterile field (see pp.190-91).
- □ Use a 14- or 16-gauge cannula (larger is better).
- □ Locate the correct insertion point: draw an imaginary line down the chest from the midpoint of the collar bone; find the second space between the ribs along this line, which will be approximately 5–8cm below the collar bone in an adult.
- □ Clean the area and inject local anesthetic under the skin (2.5-5ml 2% lidocaine if available).
- □ Insert the cannula at 90° to the skin, up to the hilt. If there is a stopper on the end of the cannula, take it off first.
- □ If there is air in the the pleural space, you will hear a hiss when the tip of the needle penetrates.
- □ Leave the cannula and needle in position. Only remove them after a chest drain is inserted.

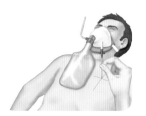

Draw lines to mark a clear insertion point for the cannula.

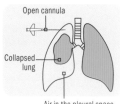

Open cannula

Collapsed lung

Air in the pleural space

Interior view: decompression for tension pneumothorax

☐ If the cannula releases blood instead of air, leave the cannula where it is, seek medical advice, and consider inserting a chest drain.

☐ You can fit a flutter valve on the end of the cannula (*see* p.196).

☐ To protect the cannula from being dislodged, you can tape it upright, surrounded by gauze (do not bend the cannula over so it is parallel with the skin).

☐ Monitor the casualty, including vital signs, to check for improvement.

☐ If the casualty does not improve, seek urgent medical advice, and consider repeating the procedure one rib space lower.

Inserting a chest drain (Seldinger technique)

Placing a chest drain involves inserting a larger tube through the side of the chest into the pleural space. This is a more invasive procedure than needle decompression and should be performed with a specific chest drain kit if one is available. Seek medical advice before attempting this procedure.

☐ Insert an IV line before you start, for use in an emergency.

☐ Position the casualty in a stable position sitting up at a 30° angle if possible.

☐ Use sterile gloves and prepare a sterile field (*see* pp.190–91).

☐ Locate the correct insertion point: on an imaginary line down the chest from the middle of the armpit in the "safe triangle" (**1**), between the pectoralis major (chest muscle) and the latissimus dorsi (the main muscle at the side of the back), above nipple level (*see* diagram).

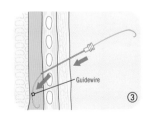

☐ Clean the area and inject local anesthetic into the skin (2.5–5ml 2% lidocaine if available).

☐ Insert the cannula just above the lower rib, angling the needle slightly toward the feet, pulling back gently on the syringe as you go.

☐ Once air or blood is released, stop pushing the needle, and advance the plastic cannula into the chest, around the outside of the needle.

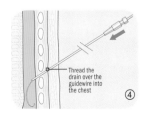

☐ Advance the cannula smoothly to its hub. Withdraw the needle, fasten the syringe onto the cannula, and pull back on the syringe. You should suck air or blood into the barrel (**2**). If none appears, start again. If it still doesn't work after three attempts, stop and seek medical advice.

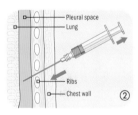

☐ When you are certain that the cannula is in the correct position, insert the guidewire from the holder through the cannula and into the chest, leaving about 15cm free (**3**). Keep hold of it.

☐ Remove the cannula (**3**), and thread the dilator over the wire through the chest wall, using a twisting motion. You may need to make a small cut in the skin with a scalpel to help with entry (**4**). If there is more than one dilator, use the smallest first and work up sequentially, holding the wire firmly throughout.

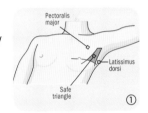

□ When the last dilator has been used and removed, thread the chest drain tube onto the wire and insert it, in a similar manner, into the chest, to a depth of 15–20cm, depending on the drain and the size of the casualty.

□ Remove the wire, and attach the tubing to a flutter valve (*see* below).

□ Insert two sutures at the entry site and tie very firmly around the chest drain tube, but not so tightly that the tube is obstructed.

□ Stick the tube to the chest with plenty of tape so it doesn't get dislodged.

□ Place a sterile dressing over the insertion site and inspect each day.

□ Monitor the casualty and vital signs, checking for improvement/deterioration.

□ If there is no improvement, seek urgent medical advice.

□ Arrange to evacuate the casualty immediately.

One-way valves for chest drains or open chest wounds

In hospitals, underwater seals are used as one-way valves, to allow air out of the chest but not back in. This method is impracticable in the wilderness and could be dangerous. A flutter valve is a better option; either from the kit or improvised.

Heimlich flutter valve

□ This is a simple, plastic flutter valve within a clear plastic casing.

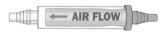

□ The valve fastens to the tubing from the chest drain and then another tube leads from the valve to a drainage bag (you could improvise with a urine drainage bag).

A Heimlich flutter valve may be included in the medical kit.

□ Make sure you connect the valve the right way round (refer to air flow arrow).

Improvised valve

□ Cut the entire large finger off a sterile rubber glove.

□ Cut a slit in the tip, and fasten the other end over the tube from the chest drain (or the needle end, when dealing with an emergency chest decompression).

□ Make a seal by winding tape firmly around the tube and glove finger.

□ Keep the end clear of obstruction.

Flutter valve for an open chest wound

□ Soak a gauze dressing swab in petroleum jelly.

□ After cleaning the wound with sterilizing fluid, place the dressing over the hole, and tape it firmly on three sides, leaving the fourth side open.

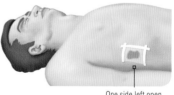

One side left open

□ This flap acts as a valve, letting air out but not back in again.

Leave one side of the dressing open to act as a flutter valve.

□ Consider inserting a chest drain through the wound, but seek medical advice first.

INCISION AND DRAINAGE OF AN ABSCESS

Hematomas (bruises) may become infected and cause abscesses (see p.165): these are relatively easy to open and drain. Abscesses that form elsewhere (on the buttocks, breasts, or perianal area) may require a more invasive approach.

☐ Apply a hot compress to help the abscess to "point" (move toward the surface).
☐ When it is near the surface, the pus may then drain from the abscess by itself—a thick gauze dressing with magnesium sulfate paste may help.
☐ Apply a sterile dressing over the site.

Larger abscesses near the skin surface

☐ Position the casualty comfortably, and explain the process. Local anesthetic is not very effective around an abscess, so warn the casualty that the procedure may be very painful.
☐ Wear sterile gloves and prepare a sterile field (see pp.190–91).
☐ Clean the area and inject local anesthetic (10ml 2% lidocaine) around the abscess, or freeze the skin with cold (cryogesic) spray—both will only partly dull pain.
☐ Use a scalpel to incise firmly over the abscess into the cavity and let the pus out (have a gauze swab ready). Incise along natural skin folds to minimize scarring.
☐ "Sweep" inside the abscess cavity, breaking down any walled-off areas with the handle of the scalpel or the end of a pair of forceps, to make sure all the pus is drained. This may cause significant pain, but be firm.

Incise firmly over the abscess.

☐ Soak a long strip of gauze in iodine.
☐ Pack the gauze into the abscess cavity until it is quite full, leaving a tail of gauze hanging out.
☐ Apply a sterile dressing, and inspect the wound daily.
☐ Remove the gauze strip on the third day. If the wound looks clean and is not leaking pus, apply a sterile dressing. If it becomes infected again, clean the cavity and repack.
☐ Give oral antibiotics (amoxicillin + clavulanate).

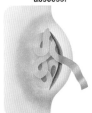

Fill the cavity with gauze soaked in iodine and leave the tip hanging out.

Deep-seated or sensitive abscesses

In the wilderness, it may not be safe to incise and drain deep abscesses or abscesses in sensitive areas. Give oral antibiotics (amoxicillin + clavulanate) and seek medical advice. If the casualty becomes unwell with a temperature, consider giving antibiotics by an IV route instead, and arrange urgent evacuation.

LOCAL ANESTHESIA:
NERVE BLOCKS AND INFILTRATION

Knowing how and when to use local anesthetic (LA) is very useful for procedures such as suturing and reducing fractures.

Lidocaine is the anesthetic agent used most often in medical kits. It is available in 1% and 2% strengths (*see below for safe volumes to inject*). For a larger dose, it is possible to mix lidocaine with epinephrine but only under direct medical guidance. Topical anesthetics such as eyedrops and gels are also useful.

Indications for local anesthesia

☐ Cleaning, suturing, stapling wounds
☐ Incising abscesses
☐ Lower limb fracture (nerve block)
☐ Damaged finger/toe (nerve block)

Cautions

☐ Allergy   ☐ Toxicity   ☐ Pain on injection

Safe dose of local anesthetics

All LAs are potentially toxic if too much is given too quickly. Lidocaine has a maximum safe dose.
For a 70kg casualty: 20ml 1% lidocaine   or   10ml 2% lidocaine

Give proportionally more for a larger casualty and less for a smaller casualty.

Toxicity

If too large a dose is given or the dose is injected directly into a blood vessel, a toxic reaction may occur.

Initial Signs	Late Signs
☐ Tingling around the mouth ☐ Blurred vision ☐ Slurred speech	☐ Low blood pressure ☐ Seizures/coma ☐ Cardiac arrest

Treatment of toxicity
☐ Stop giving the anesthetic if the casualty shows symptoms of toxicity.
☐ For seizures, consider giving diazepam 10mg intravenously (*see* pp.186–89).
☐ Treat cardiac arrest—*see* pp.46–47.

Infiltration of local anesthetic

Reducing the pain of injection
Warm the anesthetic to body temperature before injecting. When using several injections to anesthetize the area around a wound ("infiltrating" with LA), try to inject in a place that is already anesthetized by a previous injection. You can also spray the skin first with cold (cryogesic) spray or cool it with ice.

Technique

The aim is to leave a ring of LA around the wound or site.

- □ Insert an IV cannula beforehand if possible, in case the LA causes a toxic reaction.
- □ Set up sterile field (*see* pp.190–91) and use sterile gloves.
- □ Draw up the required amount of lidocaine and ask someone else to check it.
- □ Insert the needle—usually a 23g (blue) or 25g (orange)—about 5mm under the skin, and run it in up to the hub. Retract the plunger at the same time to make sure the needle hasn't entered a blood vessel (blood will appear if it has).
- □ Start injecting and pull the needle back slowly, leaving a trail of anesthetic.
- □ Continue injecting (*see* pattern in diagram) until the wound is encircled with LA.
- □ Leave for 10 minutes and check level of sensation before you start.

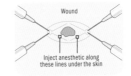

Inject anesthetic at intervals around the wound.

Femoral nerve block

Seek medical advice before performing a femoral nerve block.

Indications

- □ Fractured femur
- □ Knee trauma
- □ Lower limb fractures

Technique

- □ Prepare as you would for infiltration of LA; use a 21g (green) or 23g (blue) needle.
- □ Locate the pulse in the groin (*see* diagram), which should be in the diagonal skin crease at the top of the leg; mark a point 1cm to the side of the pulse, toward the outer thigh.
- □ Insert the needle at 90° to the skin, to a depth of 30–50mm. Retract the plunger as you go.
- □ You should feel two "pops" as the needle pierces two fibrous layers.
- □ Make sure the needle isn't in a blood vessel and slowly inject 10–15ml 1% lidocaine.
- □ If pain increases, stop injecting, pull the needle back 5mm, and try again.

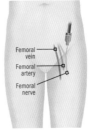

Femoral vein
Femoral artery
Femoral nerve

Location of femoral nerve

Finger and toe nerve block

NEVER use a local anesthetic solution containing epinephrine when anesthetizing a digit.

Indications

This type of block is appropriate for any wound or dislocation of the finger or toe.

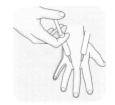

Inject on both sides of the finger or toe.

Technique

- □ Prepare as for infiltration of LA; use a 25g (orange) needle.
- □ Insert the needle on one side of the base of the finger or toe, almost through to the other side.
- □ Retract the plunger to make sure the needle has not entered a blood vessel.
- □ Inject 2–3ml 1% lidocaine as you withdraw the needle.
- □ Repeat the injection on the other side.
- □ Leave for about 10 minutes and check level of sensation.
- □ Inject more anesthetic under the skin above and below the digit, if needed.

INSERTION OF TUBES AND CATHETERS

Insertion of a nasogastric (NG) tube

Indications
☐ Persistent vomiting
☐ Loss of consciousness (to deflate stomach, to reduce vomiting risk)
☐ Distended or rigid abdomen
☐ Inability to swallow (for hydration and feeding)

When NOT to insert an NG tube
☐ If the casualty has severe facial injuries
☐ If you suspect basal skull fracture
☐ If a casualty is taking blood thinning drugs, such as warfarin, to reduce clotting. Seek medical advice before inserting an NG tube in a semi- or unconscious casualty—they may vomit and then the vomit may enter the lungs.

How to insert an NG tube
☐ Set up for a procedure (see pp.190–91). The area should be clean, but does not need to be sterile. Wear gloves.
☐ If conscious, the casualty should be sitting upright with a cup of water.
☐ Lubricate the nasogastric tube with petroleum jelly, cooking oil or something similar.
☐ Introduce the tube to the nostril, directing it toward the back of the head, not upward.
☐ As the tube passes into the nasal cavity, ask the casualty to take frequent sips of water.
☐ Continue to feed the tube in through the nose. You should start to feel it being pulled in when the casualty swallows.
☐ If the casualty gags, encourage them to keep sipping.
☐ Aim to insert 50–55cm of tube in the average-sized male. Measurements will be marked on the tube.
☐ Persistent coughing suggests that the tube has entered the lungs. If this happens, pull the tube back and try again.
☐ To check that the tube is in the correct position, suck some fluid into it. This fluid should look greenish/yellow. Test the acidity with urine dipsticks—the acid level (pH) should be LESS than 6 in most cases. If there is any doubt, do not give anything through the tube. Seek medical advice.
☐ Use tape to secure the tube to the end of the nose, then to the side of the face.
☐ Either attach a bag to the tube (such as a plastic bag or urine drainage bag) or, if you are feeding through the tube, put a stopper in the end afterwards to prevent reflux.

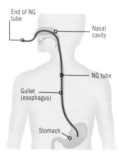

End of NG tube

Nasal cavity

NG tube

Gullet (esophagus)

Stomach

An NG tube will usually extend 45–50cm.

Insertion of a urinary catheter

Indications
☐ Casualty is conscious but can't pass urine despite full bladder
☐ Casualty is unconscious

When NOT to insert a urinary catheter
☐ In pelvic injury, with blood from the penis or vagina—
seek medical advice.

How to insert a urinary catheter into a male
☐ Set up a sterile field (see pp.190–91); use sterile gloves.
☐ Lie the casualty on his back with a bowl between his
legs—sedation may be useful (diazepam 5mg orally).
☐ Pull the foreskin back gently and clean the end of the
penis with skin-sterilizing fluid.
☐ Slowly insert local anesthetic (lidocaine) gel into the
urethra and wait for 5 minutes while it takes effect.
☐ Open the catheter packet, and locate the injection port.
You need to inject water into the balloon to stop the catheter
falling out. Read the instructions to find out how much
(usually 5–10ml) and fill a syringe with the correct amount.
☐ Hold the penis up, pulling it gently to straighten, and
insert the catheter into the urethra. Feed the catheter in
up to the hub. Urine should stream out into the bowl.
☐ Inject water into the balloon. If this is painful, make sure
the catheter is all the way in and try injecting again.
☐ Connect the catheter to the drainage bag.
☐ Return the foreskin to its normal position.
☐ Start antibiotics (such as ciprofloxacin) and evacuate.

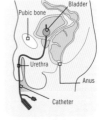

Urinary catheter in a
male—side view

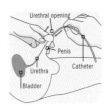

Urinary catheter in a
male—insertion

How to insert a urinary catheter into a female
The procedure is essentially the same as for a male, except
for the following:
☐ Ask a female to insert the catheter if the casualty would
prefer it.
☐ Position the casualty with her legs apart.
☐ Spread the entrance to the vagina with two fingers,
and clean the area with sterile fluid.
☐ The entrance to the urethra is just above the entrance
to the vagina (see diagram).
☐ Apply local anesthetic gel as described above.

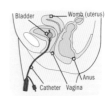

Urinary catheter in a
female—side view

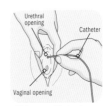

Urinary catheter in a
female—insertion

Problems
The problem you are most likely to encounter is that the catheter will not pass
into the bladder. There are several reasons this may occur. If the bladder is full
and painful, suprapubic aspiration of urine may be required (see p.202).

Suprapubic aspiration of urine

Indication
Use suprapubic aspiration if a casualty is suffering from acute retention of urine and a normal catheter cannot be used, for example in pelvic trauma if there is blood from the penis or vagina.

How to aspirate urine
☐ Set up a sterile field (see pp.190–91), and use sterile gloves.
☐ Have the casualty lying facing upward, and give sedation if necessary (diazepam 5mg orally). Position a bowl between the legs.
☐ Feel for the pubic bone (just above the base of the penis, or at the top of the vagina). The distended and painful bladder should be palpable above this point. If not, reconsider the course of action.
☐ Clean the area and infiltrate with 5ml 2% lidocaine.
☐ Use a 21-gauge (green) needle with at least a 20ml syringe (preferably 50ml). Use a cannula if there is one available.
☐ Insert the needle 2cm above the pubic bone in the midline, directing downward (see diagram); attempt to aspirate with the syringe.
☐ Urine should appear in the syringe. If it doesn't, reassess your technique. After 3 attempts, stop and seek medical advice.
☐ Once urine has appeared in the syringe, fill the syringe, disconnect it and squeeze the urine into the bowel. Reconnect the syringe to the needle or cannula, and repeat the process until no more urine comes out. The casualty should feel relieved and more comfortable.
☐ Remove the needle and apply a sterile dressing to the site.
☐ Start antibiotics (ciprofloxacin).
☐ If urine accumulates again (as it will) and the casualty still can't urinate, you may need to repeat the procedure.

Pubic bone

Bladder with urine in it

Insert the needle into the bladder above the pubic bone.

How to insert a rectal tube

Indication
The casualty needs rehydration, but oral/nasogastric/IV routes are not available.

How to insert a rectal tube
☐ Explain what you are going to do and reassure the casualty.
☐ Position the casualty on their left side—right leg drawn up and left leg straight down—on a towel placed over a plastic sheet (the procedure can be messy).
☐ Insert a lubricated urinary catheter gently into the anus. Feed it in 15cm.
☐ Tape the catheter to the leg.
☐ Connect a funnel (or a clean plastic bottle with the bottom cut-off) to the catheter, and slowly pour in approximately 100–150ml of fluid (for type of fluid, see p.184).
☐ The casualty may want to defecate, but try to dissuade them at this point. If they do pass stool, it will increase the capacity of the rectum for fluid.
☐ Run in about 50–100ml of fluid every hour as tolerated. The rectum and colon can absorb about 1.5L per day.

SPLINTS, CASTS AND SLINGS

The medical kit may contain a variety of splints for immobilizing injured limbs. If a suitable splint is not available, the environment can usually supply material for making improvised splints.

SPLINTS

General rules
- ☐ The splint should immobilize the joints above and below the fracture site.
- ☐ Pressure points should be well padded.
- ☐ Check the circulation before and after splinting.
- ☐ Remove all jewelry before applying the splint—the extremities will swell.
- ☐ Elevate the limb as far as possible after splinting.
- ☐ Check pressure points regularly.

Malleable splint

A malleable splint is a foam-covered device that can be molded, trimmed to size and used with other splints. When you trim the splint, peel back the foam, trim the aluminum underneath and cover the end with foam. Folding the splint into various shapes makes it more rigid (see diagram).

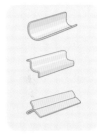

Malleable splints can be customized.

Traction splint

Traction splints are very useful for reducing and stabilizing fractures of the femur, hip and lower leg, particularly if the casualty is going to be transported. Sophisticated splints have a gauge that lets you measure the amount of traction force. These splints can be either unilateral or bilateral, the latter being more stable. When fitting a traction splint, it is vital to refer to the instructions to avoid further damage to the leg.

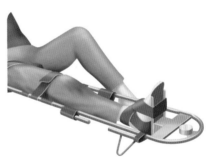

A traction splint will help to reduce a fracture, as well as immobilizing the leg or hip.

Vacuum splint

A vacuum splint is a polymer bag that contains polystyrene beads distributed between multiple compartments. There are various sizes of splints for upper limb, lower limb and whole-body immobilization. The splint is positioned around the site, and air is then sucked out with a special pump. The splint is molded to the limb or body; rigid, but comfortable. This type of splint can be left in place for up to 24 hours.

Inflatable splint

Inflatable splints are easy to carry and simpler to use than vacuum splints, but the compression caused by this type of splint can lead to pressure sores and adversely affect circulation.

Box splints

Following initial treatment, a lower limb or ankle fracture may be stabilized in a box splint. This type of splint is simple to improvise by imitating the basic design.

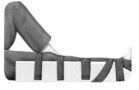

Use a manufactured box splint or make one yourself.

Improvised splints

Foam sleeping mattress Roll a foam mattress up and strap it around the limb or pelvis to make an effective and comfortable splint.

Inflatable sleeping mattress Secure an inflatable mattress around the limb or pelvis as you would a foam matress. When it is strapped on, you can inflate it to add support. Check pressure points.

Backpack frame The frame of a backpack can be adapted for use as a simple splint or as part of a traction splint.

Temporary traction splint Find a rigid pole or board that is longer than the leg. Fasten the top firmly around the top of the thigh with a broad strap and padding, and fasten a strap around the ankle, paying attention to pressure points and blood supply (*see below*). Leave the boot on if you wish (cut down if necessary) to cushion the ankle and foot. Two loops of strap or rope will fix the leg securely in place. Apply tension by fastening the ankle strap to the rigid splint, using a pulley system, and securing it (*see diagram*). Increasing the tension gradually will reduce the fracture, overcoming the thigh muscles, which may be in spasm.

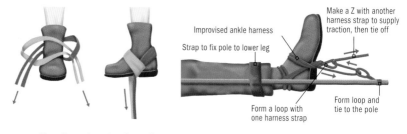

Improvised ankle harness

Strap to fix pole to lower leg

Make a Z with another harness strap to supply traction, then tie off

Form a loop with one harness strap

Form loop and tie to the pole

If you improvise a traction splint, make sure the straps are positioned correctly.

CASTS

Casts are made from synthetic-resin casting material, which is soaked in warm water and then applied to the limb before becoming rigid.

General rules for casts

☐ A cast will provide support for a fracture if immediate evacuation is not possible.

☐ Reduce the fracture/dislocation first, and check distal blood supply.

☐ Do not apply the cast against the skin—use a foam under-bandage, but not tight.

☐ Check the circulation after applying the cast and at regular intervals after that.

☐ Elevate the limb as far as possible, to reduce swelling.

☐ For recent limb fractures you should use a backslab cast, which is open on one side to allow for swelling: apply the casting material lengthwise along the back or underside of the arm or leg and use an elasticated bandage to mold the cast firmly to the limb. If the peripheral circulation worsens, loosen the elasticated bandage.

SLINGS

Use a sling in addition to a splint or cast to provide extra support for the arm after an injury. Slings may also reduce swelling and can help to reduce fractures gradually. Your medical kit may contain a triangular bandage, which is ideal for making slings, but you can use any triangular piece of cloth. To fit a broad arm sling: place the triangle of cloth against the body and fold it around the arm (**1** and **2**); tie the two ends behind the neck and pin the "tail" at the elbow (**3** and **4**).

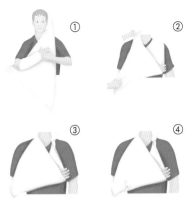

Sequence for fitting a broad arm sling

Temporary sling

To make a temporary sling, pin the bottom of the shirt or the shirt sleeve to the fabric on the upper chest, with the arm inside.

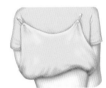

You can support the arm in a temporary sling if there is no spare material available.

High arm sling

Use a high arm sling to reduce swelling in a wrist or hand fracture. Wrap the sling as you would a typical broad arm sling (*see* above), but start with the triangular bandage on the outside of the arm, rather than the inside. One corner folds around the back and the bottom corner is pinned behind the elbow.

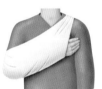

A high arm sling protects and elevates the wrist and hand.

Broad arm sling

Broad arm slings can be used for fractures and dislocations of the shoulder, clavicle and upper and lower arms, including the elbow. For information on fitting a broad arm sling, *see* above.

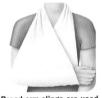

Broad arm slings are used for support in a range of fractures and dislocations.

Collar and cuff sling

Use a collar and cuff sling for a fracture of the humerus (upper arm). The weight of the lower arm may help the fracture to reduce slowly. Securing a bandage around the entire upper body, including the sling, will give extra support.

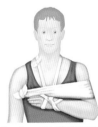

A collar and cuff sling can help to reduce fractures.

REDUCING FRACTURES AND DISLOCATIONS

"Reducing" a fracture means returning the broken ends of the bone to their normal position, in alignment. This will ease pain, increase mobility, improve the blood and nerve supply, and reduce the risk of infection in open fractures.

In the wilderness, reduction must be achieved by external manipulation. After reduction, clean and dress any wounds, especially those involving fractured bones (for more information on fractures, *see* pp.118–23), and apply splints, casts and traction as required (*see* p.203).

Fractures may be:

Undisplaced The ends of the bone are in alignment.
Displaced The ends of the bone are put out of place to either side.
Angulated The ends of the bone are at an angle to each other.
Rotated The ends are rotated in opposite directions.

| Displaced fracture | Angulated fracture | Rotated fracture |

General technique for reducing a fracture or dislocation

Aim to begin as soon as possible and before the muscles go in to spasm, which will tend to shorten the limb, making successful reduction more difficult.

☐ Find a stable position in which to work, and take usual precautions for setting up a procedure (*see* pp.190–91).
☐ The casualty has to be relaxed and have plenty of analgesia. The procedure will be very painful:
  – Sedation: diazepam 5–10mg orally
  – Analgesia: morphine 5mg IM (repeat if necessary)

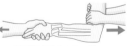

Gentle but firm traction for 5–10 minutes

☐ Use gentle but firm traction. Reduction may take 10–30 minutes, so persevere. Give more analgesia if needed (monitor vital signs though).
☐ Bones may realign with traction alone.
☐ If they do not, try using direct pressure to ease the bone ends back together (*see* diagram).

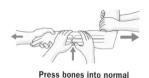

Press bones into normal position.

☐ Reassess your course of action if any of these maneuvers increase the pain significantly. Check the blood and nerve supply (*see* capillary refill time, p.181; and test sensation). You may need to splint or support the limb as it is.
☐ Apply a splint before releasing traction (*see* pp.202–203).
☐ Check blood supply, nerve supply and pressure points regularly until the casualty can be evacuated.

Specific fractures and dislocations

Dislocated shoulder

The methods below are designed for dislocations to the front. Stop if bone grating (crepitus) occurs. There may also be a fracture; support the arm in a sling.

Method 1

☐ Lie the casualty on their back. Grasp the dislocated arm around the wrist, and lift it gradually to a vertical position. Be gentle.

☐ When the arm is vertical, apply traction.

☐ Maintaining vertical traction, rotate the arm outward.

☐ If you are having difficulty, it may help reduction if you find the head of the humerus (in the armpit), and gently push it in toward the socket, maintaining traction with the other hand.

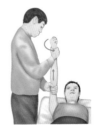

Relocating shoulder: method 1

Method 2

☐ Lie the casualty face down on a table or ledge with the dislocated arm on the outside; pad under the shoulder.

☐ Attach a 2–4kg weight to the arm, in the position shown in the diagram. Apply more weight for a large, muscular casualty and less for a casualty of a smaller build.

☐ Relaxation, traction, and reduction of the arm may take longer than 30 minutes.

☐ After relocation, fit a broad arm sling for support.

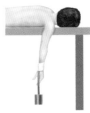

Relocating shoulder: method 2

Fracture of the humerus

Only attempt reduction of upper-arm fractures if blood and nerve supply are threatened. If you do, use the general technique described opposite. Otherwise, treat with a collar and cuff splint (wrap a bandage around the body and the sling for extra support if the casualty will be moving). In this position the fracture may reduce by itself. A cast on the upper arm will provide extra support.

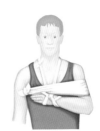

Collar and cuff splint

Elbow fractures and dislocations

When the elbow is injured, the lower arm is nearly always pushed backward through the elbow joint. The bone may be dislocated only or fractured as well. The elbow may appear bent, but should straighten after reduction.

☐ Apply traction along the line of the arm, with an assistant holding the upper arm (see illustration, left).

☐ When the muscles are relaxed, try gently to bend the arm straight.

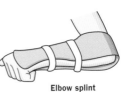

Elbow splint

☐ A clunk may indicate that the elbow has relocated.

☐ Provide support for the elbow by applying a splint (see diagram) and fitting a broad arm sling.

☐ Assess blood and nerve supply, as elbow injuries carry a high risk of damage to blood vessels and nerves.

Forearm and wrist fractures

Use the technique outlined on page 206 and immobilize with a splint that extends from the elbow down to the hand (see elbow splint diagram, previous page). Curl the hand and fingers over something soft (such as rolled-up fabric). If evacuation will take longer than a few days, the splint can be replaced with a backslab cast, which should support the arm from above elbow (held at 90°) to the hand (see diagram, right). Support the arm with a broad arm sling.

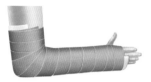

Backslab cast

Finger and toe fractures and dislocations

Reduce the fracture or dislocation quickly, before full sensation returns. If there is a delay, a ring block may be needed to reduce the pain (see p.199).

□ Pull the distal part of the finger (see diagram). You may hear a pop when it relocates. You may need to push the joint to get it back in line.

□ Tape the injured finger to an adjoining finger, putting gauze in between. If an open wound prevents buddy splinting, use a flexible finger splint molded along the back of the hand (see diagram).

□ Keep the digit immobilized for a week or so if you think the injury was a dislocation: in suspected fracture, immobilize for at least several weeks.

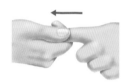

Relocating a finger

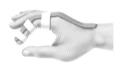

Flexible finger splint

Hip dislocation

Most often, the hip dislocates backward and leaves the leg rotated towards the midline. Relocating the hip requires very firm traction and will cause a lot of pain: use diazepam and morphine— see general technique, p.206.

□ Lie the casualty on the ground facing upward.

□ Bend the hip to 90° slowly. This will hurt.

□ Stand over the casualty with the lower leg between your legs.

□ Pull up on the lower leg behind the knee. while an assistant presses down on the casualty's pelvis to keep it from rising off the floor (**1**).

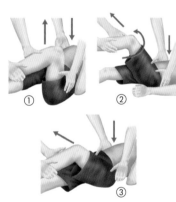

Relocating the hip

□ As the hip relocates, rotate the thigh inward (**2**), then carefully lie the leg down and strap it to the other leg (**3**). Put padding in between.

□ If there is a traction splint, gentle traction may help to keep the hip in place.

□ Do not try to relocate the hip more than three times, and carefully check blood and nerve supply after each attempt.

Femoral fracture

A traction splint is ideal for this major fracture of the thigh bone. There are many types of traction splints with different methods of application (see an example on p.203), but in general you can follow these steps. Keep in mind that other injuries may be present, so carry out a systematic evaluation (see p.33).

- □ Provide as much analgesia as required including femoral nerve block (see p.199).
- □ Try fitting the traction splint to the uninjured leg, to take measurements, before moving the injured side.
- □ Use only as much traction as is necessary to reduce the deformity—too much traction will cause further injury.
- □ Check blood and nerve supply before and after applying the splint.

If a traction splint is not available and cannot be improvised, make a simple immobilization splint by strapping boards, or something similar, down each side of the leg, from the armpit to below the feet (see illustration, above). Strap the legs together for extra support. Use plenty of padding between the splints and the leg and between the knees and ankles.

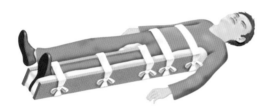

Improvised immobilization splint

Lower leg fracture

Lower leg fractures are reduced by a similar method to fractured forearms. It is possible to use a traction splint for controlled, gentle traction to reduce deformity. Either a box splint (see p.203) or a malleable splint in a U shape (see diagram) will adequately immobilize the leg. There is a risk of severe swelling, so elevate the leg. Check blood supply, which may be reduced. The casualty may need to be evacuated urgently.

Ankle fracture and dislocation

Fractures and dislocations of the ankle are often combined and are difficult to diagnose accurately. Blood and nerve supply may be compromised. Reducing the fracture and/or dislocation will require moderate force and will cause a lot of pain—use sufficient analgesia. Consider urgent evacuation.

- □ Apply traction to the foot, while an assistant holds the leg.
- □ The ankle should be in line with the lower leg, with the foot in its normal position at 90° to the lower leg.
- □ Apply a U-shaped splint (see diagram), keeping the foot at 90°.
- □ Assess blood and nerve supply. Readjust the splint if the limb is too restricted.

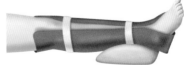

U-shaped splint

RESCUE PROCEDURES

Organizing the rapid and safe evacuation of a casualty from the wilderness is a complex process, requiring coordinated action from all concerned, including search and rescue authorities (SAR). Elements of the rescue process are also discussed on pages 14 and 87.

In order for rescue to be carried out effectively, your position must be known and communicated to the SAR team (see below), the casualty must be prepared for safe transport, landing areas need to be prepared for either a helicopter (see p.212) or a fixed wing aircraft, or other means of transport organized.

Overview

In general, a casualty should be as stable as possible prior to evacuation. Coordination with medical advisors, supplemented by whatever medical resources brought by the SAR team, should facilitate this process. Do not be reticent about calling for advice.

Try to distinguish whether evacuation is an urgent requirement or an emergency. Discuss with medical advisors and the SAR team if you are not sure. More resources may be used and perhaps more risks taken if the evacuation is deemed an emergency. Keep the SAR and medical teams updated with any change in the condition of the casualty. They may need to change their plans.

Daylight evacuation is inherently easier and safer than evacuation at night. Try to be at an accessible location during daylight, with the casualty ready to go.

While making arrangements, keep your third eye on the safety of the casualty, yourself and the rest of the expedition team. The SAR team should be experienced in these matters and should anticipate the vast majority of risks, but inform them of any special risks of which you may be aware (e.g. loose ground/ cliffs, bad weather etc.).

Emergency position determination and transmission to SAR teams

Global Positioning System (GPS) A satellite-based navigation system that automatically calculates and displays position and sometimes altitude. To be effective, it requires line-of-sight of at least 3 satellites (and 4 in order to correct errors) but usually has sight of about 10 satellites. This system has an accuracy of better than 32km under normal conditions. Signal integrity and therefore accuracy may be degraded in buildings and vehicles and in mountainous terrain. The major disadvantage is that these systems require power, which can be supplied in the wilderness from solar chargers or rechargeable portable chargers.

Personal locator beacon (PLB) Used increasingly in circumstances where the user is beyond conventional assistance. They operate on 406MHz and are detected by the Cospas-Sarsat international satellite system for SAR. When activated, all PLBs transmit a unique identification signal, and some PLBs transmit a GPS-determined position. Other types transmit an additional local homing signal on 121.5MHz. PLBs should be registered to enable full identification in the event of activation.

Emergency position-indicating radio beacon (EPIRB) Distress beacons, mainly for maritime use. These operate in a similar way to PLBs, using the same frequencies. They may be automatically activated (for instance, when immersed in water) or manually. EPIRBs should be registered to enable full identification in the event of activation.

Preparing the casualty

- **Stabilize** the casualty as effectively as possible before evacuation (*see* pp.30–33). Seek medical advice if there are any doubts. Ask for additional medical equipment from the SAR team if it will be needed (such as a spinal board, splints etc.).
- **Fully immobilize** with a semi-rigid collar on a padded rigid (spinal) board (*see* pp.178–179) if there is any suspicion of spinal injury. This may have to be compromised, depending on mode of transport.
- **Reduce, splint and immobilize all fractures** in the most effective way. Secure limbs—tape legs together, tape arms to sides—if injured or if conscious level is impaired (prevents further injury).
- **Secure all IV lines** by adhering the line to the limb in three places. If the line comes out, it may be impossible to re-insert, and immediate access for IV drugs and fluid lost.
- **Monitoring equipment** (if available) should be firmly attached to the casualty, have sufficient power and be visible at all times.
- **Chest tubes** must not be clamped or obstructed (if a Heimlich flutter valve is being used), and if an underwater seal is being used, the bottle MUST remain below the level of the casualty's chest, otherwise the fluid will drain into the chest and the casualty may arrest.
- **Oxygen** may be essential (for example, if a casualty has HAPE). Ensure that enough oxygen goes with the casualty (with a contingency) to cover the period until they reach definitive care.
- **Pain relief** should be administered and should be effective. Transporting a casualty who is injured will cause more pain, particularly if they are not properly secured.
- **Motion sickness** should be anticipated and antisickness medications given before evacuation, if possible. Being transported in a boat, helicopter, small plane or vehicle—strapped on a board in a horizontal position, with no outside view—is likely to cause nausea.
- **Documentation** of exactly what happened, when it happened, injuries to the casualty, treatment administered, previous medical history (if known), allergies, usual medications and details of next of kin should all go with the casualty.
- **Accompany the casualty** if possible. The most appropriate team member should go (not necessarily the medic—the SAR team may be better equipped and the team will still require a medic).
- **Money, credit cards, passport, insurance details and cell phone** should all accompany the casualty.
- **Food, water and a first aid kit** are also useful to include, depending on the SAR team
- **Protection** will be required for eyes/face/hands and other extremities while the helicopter lands and the casualty is loaded aboard.

Helicopter evacuation

- ☐ Evacuation by helicopter is very costly resource and should be used wisely.
- ☐ This evacuation method involves risk to the helicopter crew.
- ☐ Training exercises are invaluable; take advantage of any opportunity.
- ☐ The normal range for helicopter rescue is approximately 320km. Fixed-wing planes may be used to locate the casualty prior to helicopter approach.
- ☐ The helicopter crew are the experts. Ask their advice and then follow it.

Communicate

- ☐ Good communication with the SAR team and helicopter crew is essential to ensure coordination and convey medical information regarding the casualty.
- ☐ Direct communication with the helicopter may be possible if you have the correct equipment. Ask the SAR team about this prior to the evacuation.
- ☐ Brief your team beforehand—it will be too noisy when the helicopter is approaching/landing.
- ☐ Ask the SAR team or helicopter crew, directly if possible, about which land-to-air hand signals to use and their preferred method for marking the landing zone and indicating ground-level wind direction.

Landing zone (LZ)

- ☐ Position LZ downwind of base area if possible.
- ☐ Try to ensure the approach and departure areas are clear of any tall obstacles.
- ☐ LZ should be at least 30m x 30m—larger helicopters require larger LZs.
- ☐ Choose a site that is free of obstructions and as level as possible.
- ☐ Remove loose debris, which may become airborne when the helicopter lands.
- ☐ Inform the crew if there are any immovable obstacles, and mark them with bright clothing/fabric that is secured in position.
- ☐ Indicate ground-level wind direction with a flag or a large arrow on the ground.
- ☐ Secure all loose clothing and wear goggles/masks if on snow/sandy ground.

Approaching the helicopter

- ☐ The minimum number of people required should enter the LZ.
- ☐ Wait until signalled to approach by the pilot or crew, possibly with engines off and rotors stationary.
- ☐ Only approach from the front or sides of the helicopter, within the field of vision of the crew or pilot.
- ☐ Approach in a crouching position if the rotors are moving, in case they dip due to a gust of wind.
- ☐ If the LZ is on sloping ground, do not approach or leave from the high side. This will bring you closer to the main rotor. Use the low side only.
- ☐ Be very aware of the tail rotor, particularly with rear-loading helicopters. It may be wise to position a team member in an appropriate spot with the specific task of guiding other team members away from the area of risk.
- ☐ All team members should leave the LZ to the side prior to engine start-up and departure of the helicopter (to avoid the downdraft when the helicopter takes off).

At night

- ☐ Evacuations in the dark incur greater risk and should be avoided if possible.
- ☐ The LZ should be free of obstacles. Clear approach and departure routes.

□ A larger LZ is desirable.

□ The LZ and immovable obstacles will need to be lit in some way. Discuss the method with the SAR team or helicopter crew directly beforehand. They may require lights at each corner of the LZ and one in the middle, vehicle lights converging on the center or other combinations.

□ Wind direction should be indicated in some way.

□ Never shine any lights toward the helicopter—it will destroy the pilot's night vision, temporarily blinding them.

□ Using fires to mark the LZ may be risky because the downdraft will scatter the hot embers over a wide area. Fire is particularly risky in hot, dry climates.

Evacuation using a hoist

□ Rescue from mountainous terrain, from water or from areas where the helicopter cannot land may be undertaken using a weighted wire hoist (hi-line).

□ This is a specialist procedure. Do as the helicopter crew tell you—they are the experts.

□ A thorough briefing is required beforehand. There will be too much noise while working directly under the helicopter for anything but brief instructions.

□ A weighted line (hi-line) is dropped from the helicopter. Do not touch it until it has grounded.

□ DO NOT ATTACH THE LINE TO ANYTHING ON THE GROUND AND DO NOT LET IT GET SNAGGED ON ANYTHING OR ANYONE.

□ A crewman may descend on the wire—follow his directions.

□ A single or double strop or stretcher (litter) may be used—ensure the casualty is absolutely secured before winching up.

Special problems with airborne evacuation

□ Cramped physical space

□ Inability to monitor—vibration prevents pulse oximeters working, hampers use of stethoscope, interferes with ECG monitoring and may upset devices that measure blood pressure

□ Reduction in oxygen pressure

□ Reduced temperature

□ Noise

□ Expansion of air in pneumothoraces

□ Expansion of gastric air

□ Difficulty in performing resuscitation maneuvres if required: intubation, CPR etc.

MEDICAL SCREENING QUESTIONNAIRE

Name: ....

Date of birth and age:..........................

Occupation: ....

Address: ....

Contact Number: ....

Email: ....

Next of kin: ....

☐ Please record details of any medical conditions from which you suffer:

Specifically, have you ever suffered from:
- High blood pressure   Yes / No
- Heart attacks (myocardial infarctions/coronories)   Yes / No
- Angina   Yes / No
- Strokes (cerebral vascular accidents)   Yes / No
- Jaundice   Yes / No
- Tuberculosis   Yes / No
- Rheumatic fever   Yes / No
- Diabetes   Yes / No
- Epilepsy   Yes / No
- Asthma   Yes / No
- Depression or other mental illness   Yes / No
- Blood infections (such as hepatitis A, B or C, human immunodeficiency virus [HIV])   Yes / No
- Chronic back pain   Yes / No
- Kidney stones   Yes / No
- Cartilage/ligament injuries   Yes / No
- Musculoskeletal injuries   Yes / No
- Gynecological problems   Yes / No

☐ **If yes to any of the above, please record details:**

....
....
....

☐ Are there any inherited medical conditions in your family (please include details):

....
....

☐ Have you had any operations (please include details and dates):

....
....
....

☐ Please record any medications that you take or have taken in the past, either regularly or occasionally (please include herbal or alternative medicines):

....
....
....

☐ Are you allergic to anything (please include details of circumstances and reactions)?

....
....
....

☐ Do you smoke or drink alcohol (please include quantities)?

....
....

☐ Do you suffer from indigestion or heartburn?

....
....
....

☐ Please record details of any dental work that you may have undergone, together with an assessment of the present state of your teeth?

....
....
....

☐ Do you have any physical disabilities (please include details)?

....

....

....

☐ Please detail all immunizations you have had, together with dates (continue overleaf if necessary)?

....

....

....

....

....

☐ What is your blood group?

....

☐ What is your height?

....

☐ What is your weight?

....

☐ For insurance purposes, have you received medical advice or treatment during the previous 12 months relating to any illness, disability or condition whatsoever?

Yes / No

If yes, please detail

....

....

....

I confirm that I have answered the above questionnaire truthfully and to the best of my ability.

Signed: ....

Date: ....

From your usual family doctor

Name: ....

Practice: ....

Address and contact number

....

....

....

....

Please state how long you have been the above person's family doctor

....

I declare that to the best of my knowledge and belief the statements and particulars detailed in this questionnaire are true and complete.

Signed: ....

Date: ....

VITAL SIGNS MONITORING CHART

Temperature °C											
40 (104°F)											
39 (102°F)											
38 (100°F)											
37 (99°F)											
36 (97°F)											
35 (95°F)											
34 (93°F)											

Pulse and Blood Pressure (mmHg)

	190	180	170	160	150	140	130	120	110	100	90	80	70	60	50	40	30

Time		00:00	1:00	2:00	3:00	4:00	5:00	6:00	7:00	8:00	9:00
Glasgow Coma Score	Eyes 4										
	Eyes 3										
	Eyes 2										
	Eyes 1										
	Verbal 5										
	Verbal 4										
	Verbal 3										
	Verbal 2										
	Verbal 1										
	Motor 6										
	Motor 5										
	Motor 4										
	Motor 3										
	Motor 2										
	Motor 1										
	TOTAL										
Respiratory Rate											
Urine Output mls											

Casualty name: _____ Date: _____

Expedition name: _____ Location: _____

	10:00	11:00	12:00	13:00	14:00	15:00	16:00	17:00	18:00	19:00	20:00	21:00	22:00	23:00

MEDICAL REPORTING CHART

A detailed medical report should accompany the casualty who is being evacuated, whether by air, vehicle or physically carried. The purpose of the report is to inform the medical team about exactly what happened to the casualty, what treatment they have received and how they have progressed. It should give an indication as to possible diagnosis, and what treatments are required next.

A structured report is much easier to understand than a long rambling letter and may be read by doctors whose first language is not your own. A written report is also easier to understand than a verbal report and is an enduring record of what happened. You should keep a copy.

The information that should be covered includes:
□ Patient's name, date of birth, home address and next of kin, together with contact details
□ The main reason (illness or trauma) why the casualty is being evacuated, including circumstances and timing of events
□ The current vital signs observations, together with any observation charts already completed
□ The treatments already given and the casualty's responses, including any information from doctors previously consulted
□ All other details about the patient, including previous medical history, normal medications and allergies
□ Details of the expedition leader and the team member who was responsible for treating the casualty. These details may be important if the medical team require further information.

If you are unsure whether to include certain information, put it in rather than leave it out. The medical report must be confidential, and should only be used for the purpose of treating the casualty. It should not be passed to any third party without the express consent of the casualty.

Medical Report—Confidential	
Expedition leader:	**Name:**
Location of accident/evacuation:	**DoB:**
MAIN COMPLAINT:	**Date:**
History:	**Date of onset or incident:**
Examination:	

Vital signs: Pulse   Respiratory rate   GCS
            Blood presssure   Temperature   Urine

Treatment:

Past medical history:

High blood pressure/Angina/Heart attacks/Jaundice/TB/Rheumatic fever/Diabetes/Epilepsy/Asthma

Normal medications:

Allergies:

Next of kin:

Copies: Expedition copy   Medical team copy

Signature:

Print name:

ACUTE MOUNTAIN SICKNESS SCORE CHART

Acute Mountain Sickness (AMS) causes a variety of symptoms (see p.58), which may also be caused by a number of other problems that are common at altitude (such as upper respiratory tract infection, flu-like illnesses etc.). For this reason, making a diagnosis of AMS is problematic, but it should not be missed, as it may progress to HACE and become life-threatening.

The Lake Louise Score (LLS)* is a method of quantifying the common symptoms of AMS by setting a threshold score, above which a diagnosis of AMS is more likely. As the score increases, the severity of AMS is likely to worsen, increasing the likelihood of HACE.

One significant drawback of this scoring system is that there are no categories that specifically apply to the symptoms of HAPE, so it has no role in diagnosing HAPE (see p.58). Bear this in mind when at altitude and faced with a casualty who is obviously not well.

There are two parts to this scoring system:
□ Self-report questionnaire
□ Clinical assessment.

A diagnosis of AMS is based on:
□ A rise in altitude within the last 4 days
□ Presence of a headache **plus** one other symptom for the list opposite
□ A total score of **3 or more** if using the self-report questionnaire alone or **5 or more** if using both the self-report questionnaire and clinical assessment scores.

Indication of severity (scores from the self-report questionnaire only):
□ A score of 3–5 indicates mild AMS
□ A score of over 6 indicates severe AMS, in which case the casualty should be examined for signs of HACE.

---

* Hackett P.H., Oelz O. "The Lake Louise consensus on the definition and quantification of altitude illness." In: Sutton J.R., Coates G., Houston C.S. (Eds) *Hypoxia and Mountain Medicine*. Pergamon Press, 1992: pp.327-30.

Self-report questionnaire

Headache	No headache	0
	Mild headache	1
	Moderate headache	2
	Severe headache, incapacitating	3
Gastrointestinal symptoms	None	0
	Poor appetite or nausea	1
	Moderate nausea and/or vomiting	2
	Severe nausea and/or vomiting	3
Fatigue and/or weakness	Not tired or weak	0
	Mild fatigue/weakness	1
	Moderate fatigue/weakness	2
	Severe fatigue/weakness	3
Dizziness/ lightheadedness	Not dizzy	0
	Mild dizziness	1
	Moderate dizziness	2
	Severe dizziness, incapacitating	3
Difficulty sleeping	Slept as well as usual	0
	Did not sleep as well as usual	1
	Woke many times, poor sleep	2
	Could not sleep at all	3

Total score

Clinical assessment

Change in mental status	No change in mental status	0
	Lethargy/lassitude	1
	Disorientated/confused	2
	Stupor/semiconsciousness	3
	Coma	4
Gastrointestinal symptoms	No ataxia	0
	Maneuvres to maintain balance	1
	Steps off the line	2
	Falls down	3
Fatigue and/or weakness	Cannot stand	4
	No peripheral edema	0
	Peripheral edema at one location	1
	Peripheral edema at two or more locations	2

Total score

IMMUNIZATION GUIDE

The geographical extent of various diseases changes over time. Consult a local health agency for current recommendations. Some vaccines cannot be given to the very young or to people with particular medical problems: seek medical advice.

Diseasee	Geographical area	Immunization schedule	Duration	Notes
Cholera	Africa, South America, Far East, Indian subcontinent	Course of 2 oral doses 1 week apart complete 1 week prior to departure	2 years	The oral vaccine has superseded the less protective injectable form
Hepatitis A	India, Africa, Central and South America, Far East, Eastern Europe	1 injection 2 weeks before travel	About 1 year	A second injection 6–12 months after the first gives protection for up to 20 years
Japanese Encephalitis	Southeast and East Asia, northeast Australia, disease areas	A course of 3 injections over 30 days, finishing 1 month before travel	1-2 years	A shorter course is available but gives a shorter period of lower level protection
Meningococcal Disease (A, C, Y, W135 types)	Worldwide (particularly Sub-Saharan Africa, Middle East, India)	1 quadrivalent injection 2–3 weeks before travel	5 years	A quadrivalent vaccine protects against A, C, Y, W135 types
Poliomyelitis	Sub-Saharan Africa Indian subcontinent	1 booster dose if vaccinated more than 10 years previously	10 years	Will require 3 doses if never previously vaccinated (3 years cover)
Tetanus	Worldwide	1 booster dose if vaccinated more than 10 years previously	10 years	Will require 3 doses if never previously vaccinated
Tick-borne encephalitis	Forested areas of western and eastern Europe (including Scandinavia), Russia, China	A course of 3 injections over 5–12 months	Up to 3 years	A shorter course is available but gives a shorter period of lower level protection
Typhoid	Asia, Africa, Central and South America, Middle East	1 injection /booster 30 days before travel Oral form available	3 years	Not 100% effective so care with food/water hygiene
Rabies	Widespread, especially common in Asia, Africa, South America	Two types of vaccine available. 3 injections on day 1, 7 and 21–28 depending on type	Between 2 and 5 years, depending on vaccine type	Complete course before departure. See p.161 for post-exposure treatment even if vaccinated
Yellow fever	Sub-Saharan Africa, South America	1 injection/booster 10 days before travel	10 years	Some countries require a certificate of vaccination on entry

For factors that determine the contents of an expedition medical kit, see p.20–21.

Three medical kits are suggested here, labelled as "personal medical kit," "field medical kit" and "base medical kit." The difference between these kits is size and weight, cost and level of sophistication. Each kit is designed for a particular purpose but may be considered part of the overall medical kit resource for the whole expedition. The kit combination here would be suitable for an expedition of approximately 15–20 people and lasting 6 weeks.

Expeditions to high altitude require medications for prevention and treatment of high altitude illnesses, and there are suggested quantities here for the most important medications. Extra provision should be made, in addition to these kit lists, for prevention and treatment of endemic diseases, such as malaria. Special requirements of individual team members (such as inhalers for asthma) would also be in addition to the quantities suggested here.

The personal medical kit (**PMK**) should be carried by every team member, so must be light, compact and cover just the immediate "first aid" problems such as small wounds, blisters, headaches, insect bites, sun exposure and perhaps acute mountain sickness, if at high altitude.

The field medical kit (**FMK**) is an extension of the base medical kit and is suitable for excursions of several days into the field from the expedition base by groups of up to 6 people. It covers an increased severity of accident and medical emergency than the personal medical kit and aims to stabilize the casualty, enabling travel back to the expedition base.

The base medical kit (**BMK**) covers the comprehensive requirements of the expedition, within the design parameters discussed on pages 20–21. Its size is determined by transport considerations, cost, size of team, length of expedition, possibility of resupply and the knowledge and experience of the expedition medic.

These kit lists contain medications that may only be obtainable from a registered doctor or medical authority. It is worth investigating in good time with the relevant regulatory authorities how and where the required medical items may be sourced (see p.233).

Advanced medical equipment

There are additional items not covered by simple personal, field or base kit lists that may be considered worthy of inclusion, depending on the logistics of the expedition.

Oxygen therapy	IV fluid	Defibrillator
□ Oxygen cylinder or concentrator	□ Intravenous cannulas	□ Cardiac defibrillator
□ Pressure regulator	□ Cannula dressings	□ Pads
□ Tubing	□ Giving sets	□ Monitoring electrodes
□ Face masks of differing sizes	□ IV fluid (5–10l of Ringers/ Normal saline)	□ Service/training schedule
□ Potable hyperbaric chamber		

Using defibrillators, oxygen therapy and IV fluid requires special training, medical advice at the time of use and attention to maintaining the skills necessary to use this equipment safely.

ITEM	PMK/QTY	FMK/QTY	BMK/QTY	ITEM	PMK/QTY	FMK/QTY	BMK/QTY
FIRST AID				**ANTIBIOTICS**			
Waterproof adhesive bandages, mixed pack	1	1	2	Amoxicillin + clavulanate* 625mg		21	84
Acetaminophen* 500mg	10	50	100	Amoxicillin + clavulanate* 600mg inj			15
Ibuprofen 400mg	4	42	168	Ciprofloxacin 500mg		20	60
Diclofenac supps 100mg			10	Ceftriaxone 1g inj			10
Tramadol 100mg		30	50	Metronidazole 400mg		21	84
Codeine 30 mg		20	60	Metronidazole 500mg inj			21
Adhesive skin tape 100mm x 6mm 5 pack	1	6	6	Metronidazole 1g supp			20
Adhesive elastic strapping 2.5cm x 4.5m		2	2	Erythromycin 250mg		28	56
Adhesive elastic strapping 8cm x 5m		1	2	Doxycycline 100mg		8	16
Tough cut scissors, pair		1	1	Dicloxacillin 500mg		28	84
Foil blanket	1	1	2	Mupirocin 2% cream 30g		1	2
Hemostatic agent pack		1	2	Fucidic acid 2% cream 30g			2
Sunscreen SPF 30+	1	2	2	Mebendazole 100mg			24
Blister pack	1	2	2	Clotrimazole pessary 500mg (applicator)		1	2
EMERGENCY/ALLERGY				Clotrimazole 1% cream 20g		1	2
Atropine 600mcg inj			5	Fluconazole 50mg		7	21
Epinephrine* 1mg/1ml inj		2	10	Miconazole 2% hydrocortisone 1% cream		1	2
Prednisolone 5mg		28	56	Aciclovir 5% cream 10g			1
Hydrocortisone 100mg inj			5	**CD DRUGS (check regulations)**			
Chlorpheniramine* 10mg/1ml inj			5	Morphine 10mg/1ml inj		10	10
Chlorpheniramine* 4mg		20	60	Cyclizine 50mg/1ml inj		10	10
Loratadine 10mg		30	60	Naloxone 400mcg/1ml 3 pack			1
Nitroglycerin spray* 400mcg			1	2.5ml syringes		10	10
Furosemide 40mg			20	Blue needles 23G		10	10
Furosemide 20mg inj			10	**GUT/STOMACH**			
Bisoprolol 5mg			28	Meclozine 12.5mg			84
Diazepam 10mg inj			10	Prochloperazine 3mg (buccal prep)		50	50
Diazepam 5mg		56	56	Ondansetron 4mg (oral absorption)		10	20
Chlorpromazine 25mg inj			10	Lansoprazole 30mg			56
Chlorpromazine 25mg			56	Antacid tablets			60
Albuterol* 100mcg inhaler		1	2	Bisacodyl 5mg			20
Beclomethasone 200mcg inhaler			1	Glycerin supp			12
Dextrose gel		1	2	Laxatives (powder sachets)			30
HIGH ALTITUDE				Loperamide 2mg	5	60	60
Acetazolamide	10	56	112	Oral rehydration salts (powder sachets)		10	30
Dexamethasone 2mg		20	40	Hemorrhoidal supp with steroid			12
Nifedipine modified release 20mg			28	**EYES/EARS/NOSE/MOUTH/SKIN**			
Temazepam 20mg			28	Chloramphenicol 1% eye ointment 4g		1	2
ANALGESICS				Tetracaine 0.5% 0.5ml minims	2	5	20
Lidocaine 1% 5ml amp			20	Dexamethasone 0.1% 0.5ml minims		5	20
Lidocaine gel 6ml			4	Tropicamide 1% 0.5ml minims			20
Ethyl chloride spray		1	1	Fluroscein 2% 0.5ml minims			20
Ketoprofen gel 100mg			2	Hypromellose 0.3% 0.5ml	5		30

ITEM	PMK/QTY	FMK/QTY	BMK/QTY
EYES/EARS/NOSE/MOUTH/SKIN CONT.			
Normal saline sterile pods 20ml		10	20
Eye bath			1
Eye dressing no.16			4
Chloramphenicol 5% ear drops 10ml		1	2
Dexamethasone eye/ear drops 10ml			1
Pseudoephedrine 60mg		20	20
Throat lozenges with local anesthetic			20
Chlorhexidene 0.2% mouthwash 300ml			1
Silver nitrate cautery sticks			5
Dental repair kit			1
Hydrocortisone 1% cream 15g		1	3
Petroleum jelly 225g			1
Magnesium sulfate paste 50g			1
Calamine lotion			1
Burn dressing 20cm x 20cm		2	3
Burn bag			2
Silver sulfadiazine cream 50g		1	2
Chlorhexidene 0.015% cetrimide 0.15%		5	20
Permethrin 1% cream rinse 59ml			4
SKIN REPAIR			
2/0 silk sutures		2	6
3/0 vicryl sutures			6
Adhesive skin tape 100mm x 6mm 5 pack			10
Cyanoacrylate skin glue			4
Skin stapler			2
Staple remover			1
Occlusive skin dressing spray 100ml			1
Dry iodine antiseptic spray 100ml		1	1
DRESSINGS/SPLINTS/CASTS			
Tubular elasticated bandage 1m size B			1
Tubular elasticated bandage 1m size D		1	1
Malleable arm/leg splint		1	2
Casting pack 10.1cm x 3.6m			2
Foam underwrap			1
Leg traction splint			1
Semi-rigid adjustable neck collar		1	1
Non-adherent dressings 9.5cm x 9.5cm			10
Sterile dressings 5cm x 10cm			10
Low-adherent dressings 10cm x 10cm		10	10
Triangular bandage		1	2
Large dressings		2	6
Crepe bandage 7.5cm x 5m		1	3
Sterile gauze swabs 7.5cm x 7.5cm 5 pack		5	20

ITEM	PMK/QTY	FMK/QTY	BMK/QTY
EQUIPMENT			
Toothed forceps			1
Tweezer forceps		1	1
Artery forceps			1
Sharp/sharp scissors		1	1
Disposable scalpels		3	20
Antiseptic surgical fluid 500ml			1
Gloves nonsterile, large pair		5	20
Gloves sterile, large pair			5
Gloves sterile, medium pair			5
5ml syringes		5	20
10ml syringes		5	20
Normal saline 10ml plastic vials for inj			20
Water 10ml plastic vials for inj			20
Blue needles 23G		5	20
Green needles 21G		5	20
Injection swabs			40
Nasogastric tubes 14F			2
Foley catheters 14G and 16G			2
Drainage bag 2L			1
Heimlich flutter valve			1
Chest drain kit			1
Stethoscope			1
Aneroid sphygmomanometer			1
Large blood pressure cuff			1
Urine analysis testing strips, box of 50			1
Blood glucose testing meter			1
Guedel airways sizes 3 and 4		2	2
Nasopharygeal airways sizes 6 and 8		2	2
Pocket face mask with valve		1	1
Magnifying glass			1
Small mirror (magnifying on one side)			1
Penlight/otoscope		1	1
Digital thermometer (low-reading capable)		1	2
Duct tape, roll		1	1
Pregnancy testing kit (if women present)			2
Drug manual & wilderness medicine book			2
Monitoring and reporting charts			6
IV FLUIDS			
IV cannula fixation dressings			12
16G IV cannulae			6
18G IV cannulae			6
IV giving set			4
IV fluid (Ringer's/normal saline) 1L			8

GUIDE TO COMMONLY USED DRUGS

This table uses United States Adopted Names (USAN). If a USAN name differs from the International Nonproprietary Name (INN), as designated by the World Health Organization, the INN name is also specified.

Medicine	Indication	Dose	Cautions
Acetaminophen (INN: paracetamol)	Mild pain	1g qds	Avoid with liver disease. Not with other drugs containing acetaminophen
Acetazolamide	Treatment and prevention of AMS, HAPE, HACE	250mg every 8– 12 h	Finger tingling, altered taste, increased urine, nausea, diarrhea, headache
Acyclovir 5% cream	Cold sores (herpes)	5 times daily for 5-10 days	Start at first sign of attack. May cause stinging, dry skin. Avoid eyes
Albuterol (inhaler); (INN: salbutamol)	Asthma/wheeze	2 puffs qds or as needed	May cause tremor, fast heart rate, headache with frequent use
Amoxicillin	Ear/general infections	250-1,000mg tds	Avoid in penicillin allergy. May cause stomach upset
Amoxicillin + clavulanate (IV inj); (INN: amoxicillin + clavulanic acid)	Severe chest/ dental/gut infections	600-1,200mg IV tds	Avoid in penicillin allergy. May cause stomach upset
Amoxicillin + clavulanate (tab); (INN: amoxicillin + clavulanic acid)	Chest/dental/gut infections	375-625mg tds	Avoid in penicillin allergy. May cause stomach upset
Aspirin	Mild pain; heart attack	300-900mg qds	Avoid with indigestion, stomach ulcers, asthma
Atenolol	Antihypertensive	25-50mg od	May cause low pulse rate, low blood pressure, wheeze, fatigue, cold limbs
Atropine (IV—preferable—or IM inj)	Resuscitation	See p.29	Only for use in resuscitation
Azithromycin	Chest infections	500mg od for 3 days	May cause stomach upset, abdominal pain
Beclomethasone	Asthma/wheeze	2 puffs bd	Few short term side effects
Bisacodyl	Constipation (stimulant)	5-10mg at night	May cause abdominal cramps, griping
Buprenorphine (IM inj)	Moderate to severe pain	300-600mcg IM every 6-8 h	Avoid with respiratory depression, head injury
Buprenorphine (tab under tongue)	Moderate to severe pain	200-400mcg every 6-8 h	Avoid with respiratory depression, head injury
Ceftriaxone (IM or IV inj)	Severe chest/gut infections	1g od IM or IV	May cause stomach upset, abdominal pain
Cetirizine	Antihistamine	10mg od	Low risk of drowsiness, urinary retention, blurred vision
Chloramphenicol 0.5% eye drops	Eye infections	1 drop/2 h until infection improves. Use for 48 h	Transient stinging. Avoid prolonged use

Note: Only the most common side effects are listed. Others may occur. Always refer to the specific medicine information leaflet for further information.

Abbreviations:
amp = ampoule
bd = twice a day
IM = intramucular inj
inj = injection
IV = intravenous inj
od = once a day
pr = rectal route
qds = 4 times a day
SC = subcutaneous
supp = suppository
tds = 3 times a day

Medicine	Indication	Dose	Cautions
Chloramphenicol 5% ear drops	External ear infections	2-3 drops every 8-12 h	Local stinging. Avoid prolonged use.
Chlorpheniramine IM inj (INN: chlorphenamine)	Antihistamine, anti-allergy	10-20mg (max: 40mg in 24 h)	Drowsiness, urinary retention, blurred vision, transient low blood pressure
Chlorpheniramine (tab); (INN: chlorphenamine)	Antihistamine, anti-allergy	4mg 3-6 times a day (max: 24mg in 24 h)	Drowsiness, urinary retention, blurred vision, transient low blood pressure
Chlorpromazine (IM inj)	Severe anxiety/ psychosis	25-50mg IM 6-8 hourly	Drowsiness, low blood pressure, tremor, abnormal movements
Chlorpromazine (tab)	Severe anxiety/ psychosis	25-100mg tds	Drowsiness, low blood pressure, tremor, abnormal movements
Choline salicylate dental gel	Mouth sores	Apply bd or qds	Occasional worsening of irritation or infection—do not use for infections
Ciprofloxacin	Gut/urinary infections	250-500mg bd	Caution in epilepsy. May cause tendonitis
Clotrimazole (pessary)	Vaginal fungal infection	500mg pessary once only	A repeat dose may be required after a week
Codeine	Moderate pain	40mg every 4-6 h	Avoid with respiratory depression, head injury
Cyclizine (IM inj)	Sickness caused by morphine	50mg IM tds	May cause drowsiness. Painful injection
Dexamethasone	Treatment of AMS, HACE	8mg initially, then 4mg orally, IM or IV qds	Indigestion, abdominal discomfort
Dexamethasone 0.1% eye drops	Inflammation of the eye	3-4 drops every 4-6 h	Seek medical advice before using in a "red eye" or with signs of infection
Diazepam (IM inj)	Seizures (see p.38)	5-10mg IM, as needed	May cause drowsiness, confusion, respiratory depression
Diazepam (supp)	Seizures (see p.40)	10mg pr	May cause drowsiness, confusion, respiratory depression
Diazepam (tab)	Seizures/anxiety/ muscle spasm	5-10mg every 2 h, as needed	May cause drowsiness, confusion, respiratory depression
Diclofenac (supp)	Moderate pain	75mg bd pr	Avoid with indigestion, stomach ulcers, asthma
Diclofenac (tab)	Moderate pain	50mg tds	Avoid with indigestion, stomach ulcers, asthma
Dicloxacillin	Skin infections	250-500mg qds	Avoid in penicillin allergy. May cause stomach upset
Dihydrocodeine	Moderate pain	40mg every 4-6 h	Avoid with respiratory depression, head injury
Domperidone (supp); (outside US)	Motion sickness	30mg pr qds	Convert to oral when able
Domperidone (tab)	Motion sickness	10-20mg qds	May occasionally cause stomach cramps

Medicine	Indication	Dose	Cautions
Doxycycline	General systemic infections	100mg od or bd	Nausea, vomiting, diarrhea, abdominal upset. Not for children under 12 yrs or pregnant women
Epinephrine (IM inj)	Resuscitation, anaphylaxis	See p.29 and p.48	Only for use in resuscitation and anaphylaxis
Erythromycin	Chest/gut/ear infections	250-500mg tds	May cause stomach upset, abdominal pain
Eye and ear drops (antibiotic/steriod)	Inflammation/ infection of the outer ear or eye	2-3 drops every 6-8 h	Seek medical advice before using in a "red eye" or with signs of infection
Flumazenil	Sleeping pill overdose		
Fluorescein 2% eye drops	Staining to detect foreign bodies and eye lesions	3-4 drops once	Results in a yellow eye for several hours
Furosemide (IV inj)	Heart failure (diuretic)	20-40mg IV od	May cause low blood pressure, dizziness
Furosemide (tab)	Heart failure (diuretic)	20-40mg od	May cause low blood pressure, dizziness
Fusidic acid 2% ointment (outside the US)	Skin infections	Apply od-tds	Local irritation, itching, burning
Hydrocortisone (IM or IV inj)	Anti-allergy	100mg IM or IV tds, as needed	May cause indigestion, abdominal discomfort
Hydrocortisone 1% crea	Mild inflammatory skin disorders (eczema, bites)	Apply thinly od or bd	May cause worsening of infection if present. Avoid prolonged use
Hyoscine butylbromide (outside the US)	Antibowel spasm/ colic	10-12 qds	May cause dry mouth, blurred vision, constipation
Hyoscyamine (see also hyoscine butylbromide)	Antibowel spasm/ colic	0.15mg tds or qds	May cause dry mouth, blurred vision, constipation
Ibuprofen	Mild-moderate pain	400mg every 4-6 h	Avoid with indigestion, stomach ulcers, asthma
Lactulose	Constipation (softens stool)	15ml bd	May cause flatulance, cramps, abdominal discomfort
Lansoprazole	Indigestion, reflux	15-30mg od	May cause stomach upset, diarrhea, constipation, headache
Lidocaine (SC inj)	Local anesthetic inj	See p.198	See p.198
Loperamide	Diarrhea	4mg; then 2mg/ each loose stool. Max 16mg in 24 h	May cause abdominal cramps, dizziness, drowsiness, bloating
Loratadine	Antihistamine	10mg od	Low risk of drowsiness, urinary retention, blurred vision
Lorazepam (IV inj)	Seizures (see p.40)	2-4mg, as needed	May cause drowsiness, confusion, respiratory depression
Mebendazole	Gut worm infections	100mg bd for 3 days	May cause abdominal pain, diarrhea

Medicine	Indication	Dose	Cautions
Meclizine	Seasickness	12.5mg bd	May cause drowsiness, fatigue, blurred vision
Mefloquine	Malaria prophylaxis	250mg once a week; start 20 days before traveling	May cause abdominal upset, dizziness, insomnia, neuropsychiatric upset
Metronidazole (supp)	Gut/dental infections	1g tds pr	May cause nausea and vomiting (worse if taken with alcohol)
Metronidazole (tab)	Gut/dental infections	400mg tds	May cause nausea and vomiting (worse if taken with alcohol)
Miconazole 2% cream	Fungal foot/groin infections	Apply bd for 10 days	Local irritation, itching
Morphine (IM inj)	Severe pain	5-10mg IM every 2-4 h	Avoid with respiratory depression, head injury
Mupirocin 2%	Skin infections	Apply od-tds	Local irritation, itching, burning
Naloxone (IV inj)	Reversal of opiates in overdose	100-200mcg IV; repeat 100mcg inj every 2 minutes, as needed	May cause low or high blood pressure, heart arrhythmias, collapse. Use only under medical direction
Nifedipine	High blood pressure, treatment of HAPE	10mg immediately, then 20-30mg bd to tds (slow-release form)	Reduced blood pressure (monitor closely), headache, flushing, dizziness, fast heart rate
Nitroglycerin (patch); (INN: glyceryl trinitrate)	Angina, heart attack	1-2 patches, as needed. Replace once daily	May cause low blood pressure, flushing, headache, fast heart rate
Nitroglycerin (spray under tongue); (INN: glyceryl trinitrate)	Angina, heart attack	1-2 sprays, as needed	May cause low bp, flushes, headache, fast heart rate; use under medical direction
Ondansetron (tab under tongue)	Sea sickness	4-8mg tds	Occasionally causes constipation
Oxycodone (SC inj)	Severe pain	5-10mg SC every 4-6 h	Avoid with respiratory depression, head injury
Oxycodone (tab)	Severe pain	5-20mg every 4-6 h	Avoid with respiratory depression, head injury
Oxytocin (in the US)	Antihemorrhage from uterus (miscarriage)		Use only under the medical direction of a doctor
Oxytocin + ergometrine (outside the US)	Antihemorrhage from uterus (miscarriage)		Use only under the medical direction of a doctor
Permethrin 1% cream rinse or 5% cream	Lice, scabies, and crab infestations	Apply to whole body, let dry; wash off after 12 h	Avoid contact with eyes, broken, infected skin
Phytomenadione (vit K1) pediatric IM injection	Routine injection for newborn	1 0.2ml amp IM once	Given after birth, IM or IV
Pilocarpine 0.5%	Treatment of glaucoma	Apply qds	Headache, blurred vision
Prednisolone	Anti-allergy	10-60mg od	May cause indigestion, abdominal discomfort

Medicine	Indication	Dose	Cautions
Prochlorperazine (IM inj)	Seasickness, other causes of sickness	12.5mg IM then oral therapy 6 h later	May cause drowsiness, dry mouth, rarely tremor
Prochlorperazine (tab under tongue)	Seasickness	3mg qds	May cause drowsiness, dry mouth, rarely tremor
Prochlorperazine (tab)	Seasickness	10mg qds	May cause drowsiness, dry mouth, rarely tremor
Promethazine	Seasickness (antihistamine)	25mg every 6–8 h	Drowsiness (common); also urinary retention, dry mouth
Pseudoephedrine (tab)	Nasal decongestant	60mg qds	Anxiety, fast heart rate, difficulty sleeping
Quinine	Treatment of malaria		Only to be used under the medical direction of a doctor
Ranitidine	Severe indigestion	150mg bd	May occasionally cause diarrhea, stomach upset
Scopolamine (patch); (INN: hyoscine hydrobromide)	Seasickness	1 patch behind ear. Replace every 72 h	May cause drowsiness, blurred vision, urinary retention
Scopolamine (tab); (INN: hyoscine hydrobromide)	Seasickness	0.3mg bd	May cause drowsiness, blurred vision, urinary retention
Silver sulfadiazine 1% cream	Prophylaxis; treatment of infection in burn wounds	Apply to wound od, more frequently if discharge	Allergic reactions—itch, rash, burning sensation; apply in sterile manner
Temazepam	High altitude disorders (sleep disturbance, periodic breathing etc.)	10–20mg before sleep	Use for these indications under medical direction only. Drowsiness, confusion, amnesia
Tetracaine 0.5% eye drops	Anesthesia for the eye	3–4 drops and wait several minutes	Stings the eye for a short time
Tinidazole	Gut/dental infections, protozoal/parasite infections	500mg bd for 5–6 days	May cause nausea and vomiting (worse if taken with alcohol)
Tramadol	Moderate to severe pain	100mg every 4–6 h	Avoid with respiratory depression, head injury, epilepsy
Trimethoprim	Urinary infections	200mg bd	May cause nausea, vomiting, itching
Triamcinolone dental paste	Mouth sores	Apply bd or qds	Occasional worsening of irritation or infection—do not use for infections
Tropicamide 1% eye drops	Dilation of the pupil for examination of the retina	3–4 drops	Stinging, irritation, blurred vision

Let me not pray to be sheltered from dangers but to be fearless in facing them.
Rabindranath Tagore, 1861–1941

Despite all efforts, sometimes you may be unable to prevent a casualty from dying. This is traumatic for all concerned, especially if you know or are related to the person or have been responsible for their treatment. But remember: even in an intensive care unit, patients sometimes die despite all possible treatments. In the wilderness, remote from appropriate hospital care, you have limited treatment options and can only do your best. However, once you have accepted that the casualty will die, there is much you can do to ease the last few hours. It is a good idea to get medical advice if you are faced with someone who may be dying, and the next of kin should be informed.

Dignity Keep the casualty covered, replacing damaged or missing clothing. Obey any requests, if possible, and keep the casualty clean, as discreetly as possible.
Comfort The casualty's comfort, both physical and psychological, is imperative. Stay with the casualty continuously; make sure they know they are being cared for. Try to answer difficult questions, such as "Am I dying?," truthfully and with compassion. Make sure the casualty is comfortably positioned, warm, clean and dry. You may need comfort as well, from your team mates.
Complete relief Aim for elimination of pain and suffering—if this cannot be achieved, seek medical advice. If simple painkillers are not enough, morphine will help to reduce pain and relieve mental anguish. It can be given as an intramuscular injection or intravenously if the casualty has vascular access. Give an antinausea drug (cyclizine) at the same time, because morphine may cause vomiting. Sedation, such as diazepam, can be given as well to reduce agitation—seek advice on dose and timing.
Communicate The casualty may not be able to talk properly, but they may wish to leave a message for loved ones. Make sure they know you understand and make a written record of their dying wishes. A second witness should sign and date it.

Signs of death

Take your time when trying to establish if the casualty is dead, and preferably do it with someone else. This might be very difficult in bad weather and poor light. Make a written record of time and place of death, and both sign the declaration. There are several body functions to assess when determining death:
Breathing Check that breathing has stopped. Listen, and feel with your cheek, very carefully over the mouth and nose. There should be no sign of chest or abdominal movement. Watch for a few minutes.
Heart Feel for the pulse over the carotid (*see* p.180). Listen to the chest over the heart with your ear or use a stethoscope. There should be no noise of the heart beating. Do these assessments for several minutes, longer if you are not sure.
Pupils The pupils will be very large and will not react to a bright light being shone into them.
Painful stimulus Pain provokes no reaction. Watch the face carefully when firmly squeezing the nail beds on both hands and rubbing firmly on the center of the chest.

Mistakes when diagnosing death

Hypothermia Hypothermia may mimic death, especially if body temperature is less than 88°F (31°C). Take a rectal or oral temperature. If in any doubt, try to warm the casualty to above 88°F (31°C) and reassess. The pulse may be very slow and weak and the breathing irregular and shallow (*see* p.64).

Drugs Certain drugs, particularly sedative drugs such as benzodiazepines and opiates, may cause the casualty to have a very weak and slow pulse, with shallow breathing. Seek medical advice if there is any suspicion of drugs being involved.

What to do after the death

Take some time after the death to look after yourself and your team members.

Caring for the body

The body should be cleaned and dried. Make sure the eyes are shut (tape might be needed), the hair neat and tidy and the bladder empty (push on the lower abdomen). Bind the legs together at the ankles and interlock the fingers across the thighs. Maintain dignity by replacing clothes.

Moving the body

□ You may need to move the body to a safe place, but try to record the scene (location and photographs). Inform the local police if you have done so.

□ The body may have to be transported some distance out of the wilderness. Placing the body in a groundsheet, sleeping bag or survival bag will maintain some dignity.

□ Repatriation of the body is a matter for the local and home country authorities, the insurance company, in consultation with the next of kin.

If the body cannot be moved, carefully record the location, wrap the body securely in a ground sheet or similar (as above) and either cover it with stones or bury it in a marked grave covered with stones, to protect it from wild animals

Details to record

□ The dead person, including date of birth, address and next of kin

□ Time, place and position of death

□ Circumstances leading up to the death (accident, illness, suspicious circumstances)

□ The body, including photographs of face, distinguishing marks and injuries

□ All details of the clothing worn at the time of death—bag and keep them

□ All personal effects, which should be bagged and handed over to the authorities

□ All medical record charts

□ Statements from each of the team regarding the circumstances of the death

□ Who assessed whether the person was dead

□ Any last wishes or messages from the dead person

□ Who provided medical advice.

Informing the authorities

□ Inform the local authorities (police etc.) regarding the death and circumstances, and ask their advice regarding local procedures.

□ Inform the consulate or embassy of the dead person and ask for their help and advice.

□ It is also sensible to advise the consulates or embassies relevant to the other team members of their condition and safety.

□ Inform the authorities in the dead person's home country of the death, and of the next of kin details if you have them.

□ Inform the insurance company; they will need to plan repatriation of the body.

FURTHER RESOURCES

MEDICAL ADVICE (TELEMEDICINE)

International

IAMAT
www.iamat.org
International Society for Travel Medicine
www.istm.org

USA

High Altitude Medicine
www.high-altitude-medicine.com

MedAire/MedLink Inc.
www.medaire.com

World Clinic Inc.
www.worldclinic.com

Travellers Medical and Vaccination Centre (TMVC)
www.tmvc.com.au

Wilderness Medicine Society
www.wms.org

Wilderness Medicine Institute
www.nols.edu/wmi

Australia

The Travel Doctor
www.traveldoctor.com.au

GENERAL TRAVEL ADVICE

International

WHO International Travel and Health
www.who.int/ith

USA

US Centers for Disease Control
www.cdc.gov/travel

US State Department Travel Warnings
www.travel.state.gov/travel

Australia/New Zealand

Australian Department of Foreign Affairs and Trade
www.smartraveller.gov.au

Treksafe
www.treksafe.com.au

NZ Ministry of Foreign Affairs and Trade
www.safetravel.govt.nz

MEDICAL KIT SUPPLIERS

USA

Adventure Medical Kits
www.adventuremedicalkits.com

MedAire/MedLink Inc.
www.medaire.com

Australia/New Zealand

First Aid Kits Australia
www.firstaidkitsaustralia.com.au

Pharmacy Direct
www.pharmacydirect.co.nz

OTHER SOURCES OF INFORMATION

International

International Beacon Registration Database (IBRD)
www.406registration.com

Australia

Royal Flying Doctor Service of Australia
www.flyingdoctors.org

BOOKS

Johnson C., Anderson S.R., Dallimore J., et al. *Oxford Handbook of Expedition and Wilderness Medicine*. Oxford University Press, 2008

Duff J., Gormly P. *Pocket First Aid and Wilderness Medicine*, 9th ed. Cicerone, 2005

Auerbach P., Donner H.J. and Weiss E.A. *Field Guide to Wilderness Medicine*, 3rd ed. Mosby Elsevier, 2008

Forgey W.W. (Ed) *Wilderness Medical Society Practice Guidelines for Wilderness Emergency Care*, 5th ed. Falcon Guides, 2006

Backer H.D., Bowman W.D., Paton B.C. et al. *Wilderness First Aid; Emergency Care for Remote Locations*, 3rd ed. Jones and Bartlett Publishers, 2008

Schimelpfenig T., Safford J. *NOLS Wilderness Medicine*, 4th ed. Stackpole Books, 2006

240

ACKNOWLEDGMENTS

The illustrations inside this book are by Peter Bull and Mark Franklin.

We are indebted to many people for the opportunity to write this book, but mostly to our wives Miranda and Liz, who have yet again supported us wholeheartedly during the conception, gestation and delivery of the text. Chris Johnson deserves special mention for his painstaking review of the text and his many useful suggestions, and we are extremely grateful to him. We would also like to thank the staff at Marshall Editions, particularly Paul and Amy, who have borne our multiple revisions with fortitude and without complaint. Lastly, this book is the amalgamation of our medical experiences in the field, and, as importantly, the wealth of knowledge of the Wilderness Medicine community, to whom we give our thanks.

Spike Briggs
Campbell Mackenzie

What would the world be, once bereft
Of wet and of wilderness? Let them be left,
O let them be left, wildness and wet;
Long live the weeds and the wilderness yet

"Inversnaid" l. 13-16, Gerard Manley Hopkins, 1918